Answering the Call

Inspirational Devotionals from a Tested Paramedic

Answering the Call

Book Cover and Interior Design by Behind the Gift.
• behindthegift.com

ISBN- 978-1-64526-059-2

Printed in the United States of America.

Dedication

This book is dedicated to my old friend
Andrew James Stocks
Marine, Firefighter, Paramedic, Teacher, Soldier, and finally
N.C. State Trooper.

You died in the line of duty on September 9, 2008.
Gave your life that another might live. You are no longer
with us but your memory lives on. God bless you,
my friend. I know where you are and I'll see you again.
Until then, "Medic-7 is supersonic. We'll be there in
30-seconds!"

Forward

First Responders are always waiting. Ready and willing to sacrifice their own comfort and safety in order to protect others. I know. I was one. As a street medic I served with firefighters and police officers, emergency medical technicians and other paramedics, dedicated men and women who were willing to give their all. And together we made a profound difference. We touched, helped, counseled and saved more people than I can recall. We witnessed violence and grief. Felt victory and defeat. We saw people at their worst, rarely at their best. We laughed with many, cried with a few, saw some born, and watched others die. Over the years we carried home more pain than our minds could reasonably absorb, and many of us had to force ourselves to carry on despite the mental scars that threatened to break us down.

So after twenty years of service—of racing to calls, of plugging bleeding wounds, of starting IV's and pushing drugs, of dealing with death, and witnessing new life—I have come to the following conclusion: The most important aspect of my job was the people. My patients. My partners. My fellow First Responders. Everyone needs love. We long for the human touch. And sometimes all we really need is for another person to listen to us, or to say, "It's okay," and point us in the right direction.

5

Answering the Call

Within the pages of Answering the Call, you'll find true stories. Real situations and encounters from my days with EMS. Most are from the street, others from my personal life, but each reflects a profound moment when I heard God's voice echoing quietly in my ear.

As you read each devotional try to place yourself within the context of the story. Consider the underlying problem and the resolution at the end. Then pray for God's guidance as you work through the short series of questions that follow. Open your Bible and read the verses provided. Find out what God has to say to you. I have given you plenty of room for personal notes and prayers.

Finally, if you don't know Jesus Christ I encourage you to drop to your knees today. Confess your failures to him and ask him to become your Savior and Lord. If you already know him, I encourage you to follow him more closely. Either way, I pray that God will perform a mighty work in your life, meet you where you are, and draw ever closer to your side. And that you will respond to His voice, for sooner or later we all must decide for ourselves. There is no hiding from the truth—Jesus Christ is Lord.

"Choose for yourselves this day whom you will serve—but as for me and my household, we will serve the LORD."
Joshua 24:15

Respond!
Your life depends on it!

Here I am! I stand at the door and knock. If anyone hears my voice and opens the door, I will come
in and eat with him, and he with me.
Revelation 3:20

Imagine if you called for help and nobody responded.
How terrified would it make you feel to realize you
were all alone? Well what I'm speaking of here is eternity.
Jesus wants to come into your life. Have you heard Him
knocking? Have you responded yet? Opened the door?

"C'mon, partner, we need to go!"

"Unh uh, I'm not going."

"Right," I said with a chuckle. "Put your boots on, man. I'll
be in the truck."

"I'm serious. I wanna see the end of this game."

I gazed at my partner trying to see the humor in what
appeared to be a sick joke. "You what?"

Answering the Call

"Medic-seven?" the dispatcher exclaimed. The station radio crackled as if to emphasize the frustration in her voice. "Are you en route yet?"

"Don't answer it," my partner said leaning forward to watch a long fly ball.

"We can't just ignore it," I said. "We have to go!"

"Look, I'm not wasting my time on another silly call. It's a cardiac arrest for crying out loud. There's probably nothing we can do for the poor guy anyway."

The radio crackled again. "Medic-seven?"

"Medic-seven to dispatch," I said. "Stand by please." I turned to my partner. "Are you insane? Do you realize what you're doing?"

"Sure I do."

"Medic-seven!"

"Seven," I said keying my lapel mike. "I-I'm sorry, but you'll have to send another unit. It's my partner, he's…he's refusing to take this call."

A few seconds of uncomfortable silence passed before the radio erupted in a swarm of heated responses— the dispatcher, our supervisor, the fire department first responders already en route to the scene—everyone fighting for radio space, trying to make some sense of what they'd just heard. I glanced at my partner. He sat in front the television casually watching the game.

"I can't believe you're gonna just sit there. Someone's life is on the line."

"Relax," he said. "Sit down and watch the game. If we ignore it, it'll all just go away."

Sound ridiculous? Well don't worry, it'll never happen. First Responders are some of the most dedicated people I know. They jump into action whenever the tones sound, regardless of the weather or time of day. They do it for others, and as a result lives are saved. And yet I wonder, do these people care as much for themselves as they do for their patients? Do you?

Jesus said, "Here I am! I stand at the door and knock." He wants to come into your life. To bring you salvation, peace, and joy. Don't ignore him. Respond without delay. Because someone's life is on the line. Yours!

PRAYER

Thank you for First Responders everywhere, those
men and women who risk their own lives every day
that others might live. I pray for their safety, for
their judgment, for their salvation. They need to
care for themselves, Lord. Give them the courage
to open that door.

APPLICATION

Have you ever found yourself in that situation? Where you cried for help and no one responded? Well when it comes to eternity you have nothing to fear, for Jesus Christ is knocking at your door. Read the scripture heading again. What does he promise to do if you will open the door?

Now open your Bible and read John 14:23. What else does Christ promise to those who love him and obey his commands?

And John 3:16. What gift does Christ promise to whomsoever would believe in him?

Have you made the decision to open the door and allow the Lord Jesus Christ into your life? If not will you do so today?

BUILDING BLOCKS OF FAITH

Jesus Christ is knocking—Open the door to your heart and let Him in.

Answering the Call

JOURNAL

_____

_____

_____

_____

_____

_____

_____

_____

_____

_____

_____

_____

_____

_____

_____

_____

_____

_____

A Good Drunk

*"If you love those who love you, what reward will you
get? Are not even the tax collectors doing that?"*
Matthew 5:46

Yeah I'm a Christian, but I had me a good drunk the other
night.

No, really. I found him lying in the middle of the street,
bump on his head and a bottle of booze by his side. He
was about fifty something, dressed in simple clothes and
stinking like a sack of dirty laundry. With slurred speech
and the sweet, slushy scent of cheap alcohol lingering on
his breath, he was about as common as can get. A real
good drunk.

I chuckled. I'm a paramedic. I've seen it all before. It should
have been a simple call—pick him up, throw him on the
stretcher, and give him a ride to the ER for observation, oh,
and by the way, pray for him—but it wasn't that easy. He
became belligerent. Then he wanted to fight me. Then he
went and opened his mouth. I won't tell you what he said.
Christians don't use words like that. Or do we?

Answering the Call

I know I should have held my tongue but before I could think I flung the words right back at him. After all, he deserved it. I was only trying to help him. Right?

Perhaps, but I was wrong. Dead wrong.

You know, I've been a Christian for over thirty years, and you'd think by now I'd know better, but for me it's not that simple. I seem to make one mistake after another, failing the Lord in so many areas of my life that recently a thought has been heavy on my mind:

What does it really mean to be a Christian?

Does it mean never missing church? Attending the right Bible studies? Smiling at other people and never uttering a foul word? I believe Jesus answered my question when He said, "Love your enemies, and pray for those who persecute you." Loving those who **do not** love you is the mark of a true Christian.

"But, Lord?" I ask. "How can I love that guy?"

If I close my eyes, I can picture Jesus hanging on the cross. If I use my imagination, I can see myself kneeling at His bloody feet. But if I put aside my pride, my arrogance, and my selfish ambitions, I can imagine that man kneeling by my side—dirty clothes, stinking breath and all—and suddenly I realize this simple truth: We're both sinners. Christ died for both of us.

Answering the Call

Now imagine yourself kneeling at the cross. That gnarly piece of upright timber drips red with your savior's blood. And beside you kneels another person…that co-worker or supervisor or arrogant family member you so detest. Look at them. Do you see them? Christ died for that person, just as He died for you. So keep His commandment. Love them. It's what He called you to do.

I failed my test last Saturday night, but Jesus used that failure to teach me a valuable lesson. He showed me what it really means to be a Christian…and He used a good drunk to do it.

PRAYER

"Lord, I have rejected you and hurled insults at you, and still you love me. Help me to treat others the same way you treat me, with forgiveness, with compassion, and with unconditional Christ-like love."

APPLICATION

Jesus Christ suffered a violent and bloody death so that you might live forever, and all He really asks is that you love others in return. But some people are hard to love, and you can never predict when they will cross your path. But you can be ready for them. Take a few moments now to better prepare yourself. Start by describing a personal encounter with an offensive or unlovable person.

How did that person make you feel?

Did you respond appropriately, or in looking back do you regret your actions?

Read Matthew 5:43-48. What does Christ say about dealing with those who offend you?

Now read 1 Peter 3:9. What is the Christian told not to do?

With these scripture passages in mind, how might you prepare yourself for a similar encounter with that same person or another hard-to-love individual?

BUILDING BLOCKS OF FAITH

Love your neighbor as yourself. Do not return evil for
evil. Christ died that all might live, not just you.

JOURNAL

_____

_____

_____

_____

_____

_____

_____

_____

_____

_____

_____

_____

_____

_____

_____

_____

_____

_____

Just Say It, I Dare You!

"At the name of Jesus every knee should bow and every tongue confess, Jesus Christ is Lord."
Phil 2:9-11

When I first saw her I thought she was a ghost. She lay beneath a pile of bloody sheets, her wrists opened by a crisscrossed pattern of oozing lashes. With pasty white skin and a fixed unseeing gaze, she looked beyond help, a lost spirit in a living corpse drained of blood. Her name was Noel. She wanted to die. I knelt beside the bed and took her hand. The bones felt limp, the skin cool and dry. A weak pulse throbbed within her wrist. I aligned my face with hers. Her red-rimmed eyes seemed to peer right through me as if I weren't even there. I felt a dark, foreboding presence. Death loomed everywhere.

"Leave me," she whispered. "Can't you see I want to die?"

I dressed her wounds and explained that whether or not she agreed to the transport, I would be taking her to the hospital. The law required it. "And you need to be where people care," I added.

"No one cares."

Answering the Call

"I care. Look," I said, "come with me. My partner will give us an easy ride."

I saw her hand tremble. She shook her head.

"All we'll do is talk. I promise. Maybe even say a prayer."

She cocked her head and gazed at me. I had hit a nerve.

I wanted to tell her more—that there was someone else who really did care about her, someone who could make a real difference in her life—but I felt a dozen sets of eyes staring at the back of my head. I glanced about the room. Everyone was listening—my fellow rescue workers, the police officers, the girl's family. I suddenly felt like a coward. My tongue wouldn't move. I heard a voice within say, "Be bold, man. Just say it!" But I couldn't say it.

"Come on," I said, standing and snapping my fingers. I felt foolish, angry with myself. "Let's go."

Noel climbed out of bed and padded softly across the room. I positioned her on the stretcher, covered her with a clean sheet, and rolled her to the ambulance praying silently as I walked. *God, give me courage. Please give me courage.*

I kept my word en route to the hospital. No IV bags were spiked. No medications were pushed. All we did was talk. But as we shared I felt a growing need to tell her more. And this time we were alone. My courage grew, but still

20

Answering the Call

I felt my pulse begin to race. A hard lump grew in my throat. Why is it so difficult to say that name?

"Noel," I said, my voice low almost in a whisper. "I need to tell you something. Someone does care for you, you know."

"Who?" she exclaimed a pleading expression wrinkling her pale white face. "Please tell me."

"The Lord…" I murmured my heart racing. I could feel myself blushing. My hands began to sweat. "Jesus."

"Huh?" she said lifting a shoulder. "I didn't hear you."

I suddenly realized new strength. I felt my courage grow. I gathered myself and took a deep breath. "Jesus," I said. His name is *Jesus!*"

I saw my partner's jaw drop when he opened the rear doors of the ambulance a few moments later. For Noel looked different. Her previously washed out face appeared bright and pink. Her eyes looked focused and confident.

"What happened," Kevin said, unlocking the stretcher and pulling it from the truck.

Answering the Call

"I prayed," Noel said taking my hand, "and I know what I need to do now…I need to live. I need to tell other people about Jesus!"

It's been over five years since that night, and I haven't seen Noel since, but I know with certainty that she was transformed in the back of that ambulance, washed clean by the blood of the Lamb. And something else happened too—I was changed forever. For the first time in my life I understood the importance of boldness, of saying His name without fear. There is no other name under Heaven whereby men must be saved.

Do you know Jesus? Do you want to make a difference in someone else's life? Then say it. Be bold and just say it. Like me, you may be surprised by the power unleashed by His name.

PRAYER

"Heavenly Father, give me the courage to proclaim your Son's wonderful name, to be confident and bold, and to confess to others what I truly believe—Jesus Christ is Lord."

APPLICATION

The Bible says there is power in the name of Jesus, wonderful life-saving power. Have you ever been frightened to utter his name? Or amazed by the emotion his name seems to evoke? Describe a situation where you were forced to deal with the name, Jesus.

How did you feel at that moment? Did you feel nervous? Angry? Confused?

Read Philippians 2: 5-11. What does this passage have to say about the significance of Christ's name?

What does the Bible say should happen at the mention of his name?

Is there anyone on your heart right now? Someone you know that needs to hear the name, Jesus?

BUILDING BLOCKS OF FAITH

There is only one name under Heaven whereby men must be saved—Jesus Christ.

Answering the Call

JOURNAL

_____

_____

_____

_____

_____

_____

_____

_____

_____

_____

_____

_____

_____

_____

_____

_____

_____

_____

_____

What About Me?

"Do not love the world or anything in the world. If anyone loves the world, the love of the Father is not in him. For everything in the world—the cravings of sinful man, the lust of his eyes and the boasting of what he has and does—comes not from the Father but from the world."
1 John 2:15-16

Okay, I admit it—I love the world. I always have, it's a great place to live. But there was a time when it had me in chains, dying to get out there in it, to live a little. But my situation wouldn't allow it. And God? He never seemed to answer my question, *What about me?* So I decided to put my foot down. One of two things was going to happen: he'd talk to me, or I'd run until I dropped. I had to get his attention…

"Lord, do you hear me?" I took off down the lakeside trail shaking my fist at him as I ran. "Are you listening to me? There's so much I want to see. So many things I want to do. All of my friends are having fun. What about me?"

Silence.

Answering the Call

"Why won't you answer me? All I ever do is work. I deserve more."

More silence.

"It's not fair!"

I ran until I couldn't take another step, but still God remained silent. Finally I stopped in the middle of the trail and doubled-over, dejected and frustrated, sweating and gasping for air. Physically and emotionally I felt drained. Spiritually I was spent.

"Oh, God," I cried, tears flooding my eyes. "Where are you?"

A funny croaking sound answered me. I turned and watched a frog leap into the lake. "Very funny," I muttered. "Is that the best you can do?" Then a deer caught my eye. She lifted her head from the water's edge, glanced at me and trotted into the woods. "Hmm." A fish jumped and landed with a splash. "What is this?" I murmured. And then I noticed this dragonfly. Crazy thing buzzed past my face, landed on a small branch less than three feet away, and sat there staring at me. I felt puzzled. Was someone trying to tell me something?

Then a high-pitched mechanical sound caught my attention. Distracted I looked up. A fancy motorboat zoomed across the lake. I glanced back at the dragonfly. It sat perched on the end of the stem watching me. I felt a strange awakening in my heart. Then another boat cruised past.

Answering the Call

My face hardened again. I wanted a boat so bad I could taste it. I balled up my fist and opened my mouth to yell at God, but something stopped me—His voice. It came to me, powerful and resounding, and yet as gentle as a whisper:

You listen to me now. This world…all those things you so desperately want and can't get your hands on…don't you see? You love those things more than you love me.

My problems were still waiting for me when I got home, but something about me had changed. I ran into the woods that morning angry, frustrated and shaking my fist at God, but I walked out at peace, quietly acknowledging Him and thanking Him for my life.

Do you ever shake your fist at God? Demand your rights? Then maybe you love this world just a little too much. Put your foot down. Run out there and find Him. And when some silly bug lands on a branch in front of you and boldly stares you down, close your mouth and listen for God's voice. Then follow Him out of that deep, dark forest. He has a better life waiting for you…a life of contentment, of hope, and of joy.

PRAYER

"Heavenly Father, the cares of this world continually bring me down. Help me to stand tall today, to resist temptation, and to run a good race."

Answering the Call

APPLICATION

What is it that you cling to just a little too much? Your rights? Another person? A lifelong dream? Make a short list of the concerns in your life that would seem to tempt you most.

Read I John 2:15-16. Into what three categories does the Apostle Paul place the things of this world?

Now take the concerns you listed above and place each one in the appropriate category.

What impact do these concerns have on your daily life? On your relationship with God?

Now read Romans 12:2. What did Paul say would happen if you choose to no longer conform to the patterns of this world?

BUILDING BLOCKS OF FAITH

Contentment, hope and joy are mine when I walk by
my Savior's side.

JOURNAL

I've Realized My Calling

"I urge you to live a life worthy of the calling you have received. Be completely humble and gentle; be patient, bearing with one another in love."
Ephesians 4:1-2

"How old is she?" I asked.

"A hundred and one next month. Here's her DNR."

The nurse handed me a piece of yellow paper. I took it and studied it. It bore the familiar red "STOP" sign and the bold command: Do <u>Not</u> Resuscitate! It had been signed by a licensed physician and was well within date. I nodded. There was nothing I could do for the patient anyway.

She lay in the nursing home bed, unresponsive. Each guppy-like breath appeared to be her last. I touched her wrist. It felt warm. A weak pulse tapped beneath the dry, papery skin. I knew it was just a matter of time before it stopped. I glanced at her face. Her eyes looked empty, fixed and drained of life.

"Thank you," I said to the nurse. "We'll take good care of her."

Answering the Call

I heard sniffles as we loaded the patient onto our stretcher, muted sobs as we rolled her to the ambulance. "Goodbye," a voice said. "We love you, Hattie."

I felt a rainbow of emotions as we pulled away from the scene—sadness, wonder, guilt. The old lady's time had come and there was nothing I could do. But as I sat and watched her respirations slip away it occurred to me that I was witnessing something special, something many people never have a chance to experience—the final moments of another person's life. *What a privilege to be there, I thought, alone with Hattie in the back of my truck.* It was as if I had been invited into the inner sanctuary of something divine.

I felt a sudden yearning to reach out to her, to hold her hand and whisper in her ear. And I knew what I wanted to say. But I wondered, **can she still hear me?** They say hearing is the last sense to go.

I felt guilty as I considered what to do. Who was I to take advantage of her? She was dying. She couldn't possibly defend herself. But what if no one had ever told her? What if she had never heard the truth? This could be her only chance to hear it. It would certainly be her last.

I made my decision.

"Hattie," I said, whispering in her ear. "Can you can hear me? I just want you to know that you're not alone." I squeezed her hand. "Jesus loves you. He's with you now."

Answering the Call

To my amazement I saw a small tear well up in the corner of her eye. It rolled down her wrinkled cheek and dripped onto the folds of the pillowcase.

Does someone need you? A depressed friend or co-worker? A sister or brother who has long been on your mind? Perhaps all they need is a friend. Someone to stand by their side for that next big step in life.

Hattie didn't die en route to the hospital. We made it to the ER where she lived another forty-five minutes, clinging to life, fighting for every breath until her lungs finally gave out and the cardiac monitor traced a clean flat line. Her life ended peacefully. No advanced procedures. No heroic acts. It was a quiet death. A simple one. And I stayed with her until the end.

The paramedic's job is rarely peaceful. Almost never quiet. So for me, Hattie's passage was a special moment. I even felt as if I'd been invited to be there, to witness the final breath of another human being, a final shallow inspiration followed by a whispery, drawn out, never to be replaced breath of air. What a profound privilege, for it was at that moment I realized my true calling: to be humble and gentle, to serve others during times of greatest need, and to know without question that it's never too late, or wrong, to mention the name, Jesus.

PRAYER

"Father, help me to live in a manner worthy of my high calling, to be a humble and gentle servant, to love others and to bear their burdens whatever they may be."

Answering the Call
APPLICATION

Do you feel that God created you for a purpose? What do you believe He called you to do with your life?

Are you living a life worthy of that calling?

Reread Ephesians 4:1-2. How are you instructed to live your life? What qualities must you strive to obtain?

Now read Colossians 3:17. What does this passage tell you to do regardless of your calling?

List several steps you will now take to insure you that you live a life worthy of your calling.

BUILDING BLOCKS OF FAITH

A Christian must clothe himself with humility, gentleness and patience, bearing with other believers, for this is the will of God.

JOURNAL

We Must Walk By Faith!

"We live by faith, not by sight."
II Corinthians 5:7

I found the bus parked on the side of the road. A small crowd stood to one side, shocked expressions on their faces. I climbed aboard and found my patient sitting in the aisle on a pile of broken glass, her hands pressed to her forehead, arms and lap stained with blood. She might have been angry—cursing and shaking her fist at the foolhardy teenagers whom had reportedly heaved a rock at the bus, shattering the window and hitting her in the head. But she didn't seem upset.

She took a deep breath, told me her name, and then quietly submitted as I lowered her hands to examine the wound. And it was deep—a three inch gash above her right eyebrow. A golf ball sized hematoma had already formed. Her eyelid looked swollen, discolored and wet.

"It could be worse," I said, taking a wad of water soaked gauze and gently cleansing the site. "But you're going to need stitches."

38

Answering the Call

"There's glass in my eye," she said. "I can't open it."

"Don't try."

I finished washing the wound and dressed it with fresh gauze, careful to cover both of her eyes to prevent unintentional movement.

"Now," I said taking her hands, "stand up and follow me. My partner has the stretcher at the bottom of the steps."

I saw her face draw up tight. "But I can't see. How can I—"

"Lisa. Trust me."

"But—"

"Think of it as a faith walk."

Her face relaxed. She nodded as if she understood the meaning of the scripture…to walk by faith means a willingness to close one's eyes. To trust in the Lord, with all of one's heart.

I helped her stand and then backed down the aisle, coaxing her with quiet words of encouragement. Her first few steps seemed timid, unsure, but her faith seemed to grow as we gained momentum. Together we walked down the steps, through the door, and outside into the humid night air.

Answering the Call

The back of the ambulance was cool and bright. I checked her vital signs and started an IV. We made small talk about the event, about her wounds, and eventually the conversation turned to faith.

"You're a Christian, aren't you?" she said. It was more of a statement than a question.

"Yes, I am."

"Will you pray for me?"

Now I wish I could say I'm a saint, but I'm not. And I wish I could tell you I pray with every patient in the back of my ambulance, but I don't. I've argued with many, fought with a few, and battled my own prejudices more times than I can remember. "But her question? It reminded me...I had a job to do."

"Of course I'll pray with you," I said.

So we prayed. Two people from different worlds meeting in the most unlikely of circumstances, holding hands and praying as if we'd known each other for years. They say God works in strange ways; I see it more as creative brilliance. His love breaks down barriers, shatters human defenses. It brings people together who might otherwise never meet.

"You know what's fascinating?" I said when I raised my head from prayer. "You haven't even seen me yet and still, you trust me."

Answering the Call

She nodded. Then smiled. I couldn't see beneath the bloody bandages, but I'm sure her eyes twinkled.

"We live by faith," she murmured, "not by sight."

Amen to that.

Are you facing a challenge? A wall too high to climb? Tell the Lord. Trust Him. And then take hold of His gentle hands and follow Him toward the light.

PRAYER

"Lord, help me to follow you, to trust you with all of my heart, and to walk by faith instead of relying on my own limited judgment."

APPLICATION

The First Responders in your community—the paramedics, the police officers and firefighters—share a fraternal faith, a trust that is best described as 'watching the other man's back.' They must, for it's a necessary part of the job. But in everyday life it can be difficult to find another person you trust with all you have. Can you describe a situation where you were compelled to trust another person with something precious, like say your life, or that of a family member or close friend?

How did it make you feel to know that one of your most valuable possessions was in another person's hands?

Read Deuteronomy 31:6 and Joshua 1:5. What do these scriptures say regarding God's intention to always watch your back?

How might these promises change your daily life? Your commitment to prayer?

43

BUILDING BLOCKS OF FAITH

Trust the Lord, acknowledge Him in all you do, and He will show you which path to walk.

JOURNAL

_____

_____

_____

_____

_____

_____

_____

_____

_____

_____

_____

_____

_____

_____

_____

_____

Clear in Any Language

Finally, all of you, live in harmony with one another; be sympathetic, love as brothers, be compassionate and humble.
1 Peter 3:8

I admit it. I didn't want to touch the guy. He sat on the edge of the bed with his leg elevated. His knee looked swollen and red with infection. Yellow pus oozed from between the stitches. My nose drew up. I felt my guts tighten. I swallowed the bile in the back of my throat and approached him.

"Hey," I said, certain I knew the answer he would give. "Do you speak English?"

He shook his head. I saw fear in his eyes.

I should have introduced myself, made an attempt at friendliness and tried to gain his trust, but I didn't. I performed a rough assessment careful to keep my gloved hands as far away from the festering wound as possible.

45

Answering the Call

After checking his vital signs I sent my partner to the truck for the stretcher and quickly wrapped the wound with dressings. I just wanted to get the job done. Get out. Get on to something else. *After all,* I thought, *this guy doesn't deserve my help.* He's just like all the rest of them. He's using us. Trespassing. He doesn't belong here!

My patient seemed to read my mind. He murmured something and tried to stand, but he didn't get far. He grimaced. His red-rimmed eyes filled with tears. He fell back onto the dirty sheets and squeezed his thigh, crying. I couldn't understand what he said but it didn't matter. The pain on his face would have been clear in any language. He needed help.

Suddenly it occurred to me how selfish I had been. I wasn't acting like a Christian at all. There was no kindness in my voice, not a trace of compassion in my touch. I paused and stared deep into his panicked eyes and instantly my vision cleared. No longer was I dealing with an illegal alien. I was helping my fellow man. He had a handsome face and strong brown eyes. He probably even had a proud name.

"My God," I whispered, "forgive me."

I felt new warmth flow through me. I felt stronger, more compassionate. I slowed down, properly dressed his wound, and then stopped and looked him in the eyes.

"Amigo—" I tapped my chest. Shook my head. "I'm sorry, friend. My name is Pat."

Answering the Call

His eyes widened. The corners of his mouth drew up in a timid smile. "Si," he said. A gentle nod. "Me llamo German…" *(my name is Hermaan)*

We had a short ride to the ER. I rechecked his wound, started an IV, and then sat back and continued my feeble attempt at communication. I stuttered a little, shrugged a lot, and occasionally shook my head. A couple of times I even laughed. So did Hermaan. He still hurt—I could tell by the way he clinched his teeth every time the ambulance hit a bump—but his fear and distrust had vanished.

As we arrived at the hospital it occurred to me that my patient and I had hit it off. He still smelled, his wound still reeked and his clothes still stank, but I no longer cared. I'd made a new friend, and in doing so healed a lifetime of bitterness and distrust.

PRAYER

"Lord, thank you for loving me. Help me to be kind
and compassionate, and to always love my fellow
man regardless of his background or race."

Answering the Call

APPLICATION

If you are like most people, you struggle with a certain amount of prejudice. Will you be honest with yourself and admit a prejudice you hold toward another race or group of people?

Have you ever been forced to deal with that prejudice through direct encounter with another individual? If so, how did you feel at the time? Superior to the other person? Inferior? Did you experience a certain amount of distrust?

Reread the scripture passage again, 1 Peter 3:8. How does God expect you to treat that individual?

Now read Ephesians 4:32 to 5:2. Whom do the scriptures say you should imitate whenever you deal with other people? How are you supposed to do it?

What exactly does this passage indicate that Jesus Christ did for you? How might this knowledge change your prejudice toward that person or group of people?

BUILDING BLOCKS OF FAITH

The fruit of the Holy Spirit are love, joy, peace, patience,
goodness, kindness, faithfulness, gentleness and self-control.

JOURNAL

_____

_____

_____

_____

_____

_____

_____

_____

_____

_____

_____

_____

_____

_____

_____

_____

_____

_____

Fight for Position. Fight!

The LORD is my shepherd; I shall not want. He ma-
keth me to lie down in green pastures: He leadeth me
beside the still waters. He restoreth my soul.
Psalm 23:1-3

Total loyalty. Total trust. Total dependence.

Every time I read Psalm 23 I imagine a flock of sheep fighting for position. They push, they struggle, each trying his best to draw close to the shepherd's leg while an army of angry red eyes glares at them from the darkness. They hear vicious growling, angry pawing, and the relentless snarling of hungry creatures eager to tear at their soft pink flesh. But the flock remains safe. It grazes in perfect peace, totally aware of the dangers, but secure in the knowledge that the shepherd is keeping watch, his rod and staff in hand.

What a beautiful image. No scripture encourages me more. But when I realize that it was written for me, about me, I'm humbled. For I am one of those lost sheep. We are his flock.

Answering the Call

We live in a dangerous world, surrounded by terror. Evil men plot against us, to maim, kill, and destroy our way of life. Follow the world, stray off of God's chosen path, and, in the end, you will be dragged down a road of destruction with the eternal darkness of hell at the end. Yes, death is all around us and it can strike at any moment. So what are we to do? Where is our shepherd? Who will raise his staff to fight on our behalf?

As I reflected on the tragedy of 9/11 this week, that question came to mind. On that terrible day 2,983 of our brothers and sisters felt the wolves' teeth tear into their flesh. Evil attacked. And innocent people died. A cruel picture? You bet it is, but it's one we must never forget. If we learn nothing else from their needless sacrifice, let us learn this: Like sheep, we are all vulnerable. We need a shepherd. We need salvation from this lost and dying world.

None of us knows when our time will come, so before you go to work, to class or to bed, ask the Lord Jesus Christ to walk into your life. He is the Great Shepherd, your rock and your fortress against the dangers of this world.

And when the darkness closes in, when the killing wolves attack, draw as close to Him as you can. Fight for position. Fight! And when your time comes—when it's your turn to walk through the Valley of the Shadow of Death—your shepherd will be standing by your side. His rod and his staff, they will protect you!

PRAYER

The people who went to work that tragic morning, and all of the firefighters, police officers and paramedics who died in the line of duty, none of them realized their lives would be demanded of them that day. Help us to learn from their misfortune, to be aware of the dangers surrounding us, and to draw as close to you as we can. None of us knows when our time will come.

Answering the Call

APPLICATION

Do you remember how you felt on the morning of 9/11/2001 when America fell under attack? Did you feel frightened? Uncertain? Could you sense the hungry wolves staring at you from the darkness? Describe the way you felt that morning.

Read Psalm 23…Try to envision the scene. Can you see the meadow? The cool blue waters? Can you imagine the sheep gathered around the shepherd, terrified, fighting for position to draw as close to his legs as possible as the fiery red eyes peer at them from the darkness? And the shepherd? His strong hand tightly gripping his wooden staff, no trace of fear on his face. Do the sheep appear safe by his side? Describe how this passage makes you feel.

Now imagine that you are one of those sheep. How would you feel if the shepherd suddenly abandoned you leaving you alone to face the hungry wolves?

Answering the Call

Read Deuteronomy 31:1-6. What did Moses promise the Israelites regarding the Lord their God?

Now read Joshua 1:1-5. What was God's promise to Joshua?

Also read Matthew 28:16-20. How long did Jesus promise that He would stay with His disciples?

Jesus is the good shepherd (John 10:11). If you are following him you have nothing to fear. How might this change the way you respond the next time you feel frightened?

BUILDING BLOCKS OF FAITH

God knows the day, the hour, the exact moment your life will end. And after that comes eternity. Do you know Jesus? Have you received His gift of everlasting life?

Answering the Call

JOURNAL

_____

_____

_____

_____

_____

_____

_____

_____

_____

_____

_____

_____

_____

_____

_____

_____

_____

_____

_____

_____

_____

_____

A Real Miracle

He performs wonders that cannot be fathomed,
miracles that cannot be counted.
Job 5:9

My job is unpredictable, out of control at times, and just occasionally I need a little help. But sometimes I need a real miracle. My last call was one of those times.

"Excuse me. Move please. Hey! I said, move!"

My partner, Larry, pushed through the crowd of nervous onlookers. He carried an orange airway bag over his shoulder; I carried a ton of uncertainty in my heart. Three men dressed in bunker pants and navy blue fire department tee shirts knelt over a small inert body in the middle of the street. Fire Captain David Young looked up at me and grimaced. "Boy, am I glad to see you guys. His airway's as tight as a plugged pipe."

"How long has he been down?" I asked, glancing at the child's face. The small brown eyes appeared lifeless, the lips the color of a purple Popsicle.

Answering the Call

"Six or eight minutes," Young responded. "Maybe more." I sighed, kneeling beside my patient. Larry handed me a bag-valve-mask resuscitator. I placed it over the boy's mouth and nose and gave the bag a squeeze. I hoped to see his chest rise as his tiny lungs filled with air, but it didn't. The air squeaked out of the sides of the mask instead of flowing down his throat and into his lungs. His airway was blocked.

Larry handed me a laryngoscope. I inserted the tip of the blade into the child's mouth and lifted his tongue. The fiber-optic bulb lit the back of his throat all the way to the vocal cords. "Hmm," I murmured. "Not good."

"What is it," Larry said. "See anything?"

"Something's blocking his airway, but I can't see it. Quick," I said, holding out my hand and snapping my fingers. "Let's tube him." Larry placed a clear, slender endotracheal tube into my hand. I inserted it into the boy's throat and passed the tip through the vocal cords, but it stopped short as if hitting a wall. "Something's down there," I said withdrawing the tube, "but I don't see it. Do some more thrusts."

Nobody moved.

"Come on," I shouted. "Do it!"

One of the firefighters straddled the child, placed his hands on the boy's abdomen, and gave five, quick upward thrusts. I tried again. The tube stopped short. I felt myself begin to panic. The child's airway was completely blocked. He was *going* to die. I needed a miracle.

Answering the Call

What does that scripture say? He performs wonders no man can understand? Miracles too numerous to count?

"Jesus," I whispered. "Help me."

I tried again. No luck. My heart broke.

"Let's go!"

I picked up the boy and ran for the ambulance. I climbed into the back of the truck and placed him on the stretcher. Larry climbed in behind me and slammed the doors. The truck began to move. The siren wailed. We tried again to clear the little boy's airway, first using the Heimlich maneuver, then another ET tube. No change. There was nothing more we could do.

"Oh, Lord," I cried, "Please help us!"

Suddenly I felt a heavy jolt as the truck hit a deep pothole. The rear end jumped up then landed hard on one side and lurched upward again. I lost my balance and fell to the floor. I wanted to curse, to shout out in anger and frustration. *Why did you fail me, God? Why?*

"Hey," Larry shouted. "There it is!"

He reached into the boy's mouth and removed a small round object. He wiped away a layer of creamy white saliva and held it up for me to see.

"It's a grape!"

Answering the Call

Do you believe in miracles? I sure do. That little boy choked on that grape and should have died. Fifteen minutes without air and life as we know it is all but impossible…but not with God. By the time we left the ER the boy was wide-awake and sitting up with his family, as healthy looking a child as I had ever seen. Yes, I believe in miracles. Our God is real.

Don't you ever give up! No matter how huge the mountain you face, God is bigger. And He still performs wonders, the likes of which no man could ever imagine.

PRAYER

"Lord, my life is unpredictable. Sometimes out of control. Help me to remember that you are still in charge, always ready to handle even my toughest problems."

Answering the Call

APPLICATION

Have you ever been in a situation where you felt totally out of control? When there was nothing left to do but cry for help? Describe that situation.

How did you handle it? Did you pray? Curse? Ask another person for help?

Read Mark 4:35-41. What did Jesus do when his disciples cried out to him for help?

Now read Matthew 14:23-32. What did Jesus do when Peter began to sink?

According to Job 5:9, what kind of wonders does God perform?

Next time you find yourself out of control, how will you respond differently than the previous time?

BUILDING BLOCKS OF FAITH

He performs wonders that cannot be fathomed.

JOURNAL

A Second Chance

Jesus said to her, "I am the resurrection and the life.
He who believes in me will live, even though he dies; and
whoever lives and believes in me will never die.
Do you believe this?"
John 11:25

I thought I'd been had. A group of old men sat in rocking chairs on the front porch of the retirement home. Their aged faces reflected serenity. Their expressions revealed not a care in the world. I stepped onto the porch and cleared my throat. No one spoke or greeted me. They hardly seemed to notice me.

"Excuse me," I said feeling somewhat confused, quite certain that my EMS uniform would have been enough to announce the purpose of my visit. "Did you gentlemen call 9-1-1?"

"Sure, sure," one of the men said. "We called you."

"Well?" I said with a chuckle. "What can we do for you, sir?"

Answering the Call

"I think Harold's dead." He pointed across the porch. "Stopped breathing a few minutes ago."

"What?" I hurried over to check Harold's status. Sure enough, the gray-haired old man sat motionless in his rocker, his head slumped against the shoulder of one of his buddies as if asleep. I saw no sign of life, no movement at all. I touched his neck and felt for a pulse. Nothing.

"Uh, Andy?" I glanced at my partner. "I believe he's right."

There's one thing for sure—death awaits us all. But what comes after that? Eternal life? Hell? Nothing? Jesus said whoever believes in Him would live and never die.

Andy powered up the defibrillator unit. I grabbed the old man by the arms, slid him to the floor and ripped open the front of his shirt. Buttons flew. Fabric tore. Andy handed me the paddles. I placed them on his chest. I glanced at the monitor. A squiggly green line traced across the screen.

"Okay, we've got V-Fib," I said. "We can handle that."

Andy switched the unit to DEFIB and pushed the charge button. The unit began to whine. The low-toned whistle built quickly into a high-pitched shrill.

"Okay," Andy said, the capacitor fully charged. "Light him up."

"Clear!"

Answering the Call

Andy backed away. I straightened my arms, pushed the paddles firmly against Harold's bony chest, and delivered the shock. Two hundred watt-seconds of electricity discharged into the old man's body. His back arched. His muscles jerked. And then suddenly, to my amazement, he opened his eyes. He looked about briefly as if trying to gain his bearings, and then turned and gazed at me.

"Who are you?"

"Sir," I said, trying to hide my astonishment. "I'm a paramedic."

"What are you doing?"

"You were dead, Harold," one of the old men shouted. "These boys saved your life."

"They did? Well, ain't that something?" Harold sat up and rubbed his chin. "Thanks, fellas. Looks like I got me a second chance."

God has offered you a second chance too. A priceless gift called everlasting life. Have you accepted it? Will you?

Harold died that cool autumn evening but apparently God wasn't finished with him. He sent Andy and me, and by the delivery of a single shock of electricity He gave Harold a second shot at life. You may not be as fortunate as Harold was, so don't delay that decision. Say yes to God's Son, Jesus Christ. He is your second chance.

PRAYER

"Thank you, Heavenly Father, for gift of everlasting life, and for using Harold to remind me of the importance of telling others."

Answering the Call

APPLICATION

In Ecclesiastes 3:1, King Solomon wrote, "There is a time for everything, and a season for every activity under heaven..." Read verses 2-8. What does this passage tell you about death?

Death is inevitable. The question then is what happens next? The Prophet Daniel wrote, "everyone whose name is found written in the book will be delivered. Multitudes who sleep in the dust of the earth will awake: some to everlasting life, others to shame and everlasting contempt." (See Daniel 12:1-2). If you could choose between the two, would you choose everlasting life or everlasting contempt?

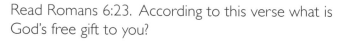

Answering the Call

Read Romans 6:23. According to this verse what is God's free gift to you?

Now read Romans 10: 9-13. What must a person do in order to receive this free gift?

You do not know when your time will come, but you can experience everlasting life. Will you now accept God's free gift of everlasting life through Jesus Christ?

BUILDING BLOCKS OF FAITH

Be vigilant. Keep watch. No man knows when his hour
will come.

JOURNAL

Power for the Weak

Do you not know? Have you not heard? The LORD
is the everlasting God, the Creator of the ends of the
earth. He will not grow tired or weary, and His understanding no one can fathom. He gives strength to the
weary and increases the power of the weak.
Isaiah 40:28-29

My youngest son was fourteen at the time, healthy, safe,
and getting himself ready for school when my final call of
the night shift began.

"EMS report for medic-seven," the dispatcher said.
"Possible suicide."

Terrible images flooded my mind as I ran for my truck.
Slashed wrists. Gunshot wounds. Horrific expressions of
self-inflicted death.

"You can handle this," I told myself. "It's just another call."

But it wasn't. We found her lying at the base of a carpeted
staircase—a fourteen-year-old girl with no sign of life.

Her eyes bulged. Her face looked puffy and blue. A collar
of swollen red skin encircled her neck.

Answering the Call

"She hung herself," a police officer explained. "Her little sister found her. Cut her down and ran back to bed. Can you believe it? Poor kid didn't know what else to do."

Have you ever felt the harshness of life slap you in the face? Witnessed death or cruelty, or shared in the suffering of a loved one or friend?

I wanted to cry but I couldn't. My defense mechanisms worked too well. I glanced around the room. Other faces reflected anger, pain and disbelief, but I felt nothing. No sorrow. No pity. Just numbness.

"You can handle it," I whispered. "It's just another call."

Weeks passed, then months. My life went on as usual. Then one day another crisis jolted me, this time in **my** home. I'd lost someone I loved, and I didn't know what to do.

My defense mechanisms went to work again. I prepared myself for the worst.

"You can handle it," I told myself. "It's just another call."

But this time I was wrong. Like a pressure cooker blowing off steam, I exploded. I broke down in a fit of uncontrolled grief while my wife, my sons and my in-laws watched, bewildered by my sudden burst of emotion.

Embarrassment could not begin to explain the humiliation I felt that day. But I couldn't help myself, it just happened. Fifteen years of pent up frustration and anger, grief and

Answering the Call

hopelessness, sorrow and death—they all finally surfaced, and with them a tidal wave of emotion that truly rocked my world. And for the first time in my life I understood the meaning of the scripture: *He gives strength to the weary and increases the power of the weak.*

"Give me strength, Lord, I'm weary. Give me power, I'm so weak."

My family survived that crisis. God poured out His mercy on us...especially on me. I still find myself crying at times when the harsh realities of life slap me in the face, but I handle the pain better now. I'm stronger, more resilient, better equipped to let it all go.

When you feel tired and weary, unable to manage the stress in your life, ask God for the strength to make it through. The power to push on when you feel you've reached your end.

PRAYER

"Lord, you have shown me that I can't make it own
my own. Thank you for giving me new strength,
and for helping me day by day."

APPLICATION

When facing the trials of life it is often difficult to remain focused, to hold one's head high and trust God with all of your heart. Describe a situation where you found yourself overwhelmed, unable to cope with a problem or insurmountable task.

Did you feel stronger because of the challenge or tired and weary due to your lack of situational control?

Did your emotions get the better of you? How did you feel? Frightened? Discouraged? Take a moment to describe your feelings at that moment.

Read Isaiah 40:28-29. What does this passage mean to you? Who provides strength to the weary? Power to the weak?

Answering the Call

Now read Psalm 90:2. What does the Psalm tell you about God?

Also read Isaiah 40:26. Why is it that not a single star is missing? Go outside and study the sky at twilight. Watch the stars appear one by one as the sky turns black. Who is it that Isaiah tells us watches over this event every night?

Next time you feel tired or weary what will you do differently? Remember, God gives strength to the weary and increases the power of the weak.

BUILDING BLOCKS OF FAITH

God's people shall run and not grow weary. They shall walk and not faint. He gives strength to the weary and power to His saints.

Answering the Call

JOURNAL

_____

_____

_____

_____

_____

_____

_____

_____

_____

_____

_____

_____

_____

_____

_____

_____

_____

_____

The Armor of God

Finally, be strong in the Lord and in his mighty power. Put on the full armor of God so that you can take your stand against the devil's schemes. For our struggle is not against flesh and blood, but against the rulers, against the authorities, against the powers of this dark world and against the spiritual forces of evil in the heavenly realms.
Ephesians 6:10-12

It's my routine each night as I drive to work: Leave the house, drive north 2.5 miles, and then hang a left. The highway is long and straight, and for fifteen miles I'm alone with my thoughts. I use that time to think. And to pray. "Help me to be a good paramedic. Please don't let me hurt anyone tonight. And, Lord, please help me to be a gentleman."

That night I clocked in at 7:00 p.m. and right away the calls began. Tough calls. The kind that make me wonder why I still do this job? One patient lied to my face, another spit at me. A belligerent female cursed at me, blamed me for her plight in life and then accused me of racism.

78

Answering the Call

The hours ticked away; the calls continued to come. Exhausted and weary from the workload, I grew frustrated by the onslaught of personal insults. But I remained in control, presented myself as a gentleman.

Until 4:00 a.m.

The armor of God. It protects us from the unexpected, those difficult moments when our faith is tested most.

I found her vehicle atop a grove of broken pines. Prickly vines tore at my skin as I climbed down the embankment and looked the shattered side window into her car. "Hello," I said, scanning my patient for major injuries. "My name's Pat. What's yours?"

"Get me out of here," she shouted.

"Well we will," I said, "but first tell me, are you breathing okay? Are you hurt?"

"Shut up and get me out here," she shouted. "Now!"

Ever find yourself blindsided, hit by a situation that pushed you over the edge?

I bit my tongue and continued my assessment. Trauma victims sometimes speak irrationally, I knew, and say things they don't mean. But I found no major injuries or any reason for her rude belligerence.

I explained the situation to her as the firefighters approached the car. She continued to fuss as they pulled open her door, continued to gripe as we immobilized her to a spine board and carried her up the hill.

She fought me the whole way to the hospital, pulling at her bindings and yelling for me to cut her loose. I tried to remain patient, continued to help. I even stabilized her on a particularly rough section of road—grabbed her belt and held on tight to keep her from rolling as the truck rocked side to side—but she rejected my act of kindness and turned it into something else.

"Don't you do it," she threatened. "Don't you dare touch me like that!"

"What!" I released her belt. "You're accusing me of abusing **you**?"

I couldn't believe it. How much abuse is a man supposed to take? I'd already been reviled, and spit at, and torn to pieces by a tangle of gnarly thorns, but this? Enough was enough. She started to respond to the question but I would not allow it. "Shut up," I said, pushing away and moving as far from her as the ambulance walls would allow.

"What?" she said. A look of incredulity crossed her face. "What did you say to me?"

"I SAID, SHUT UP!"

And she did. She remained as passive as a lamb for the rest of the ride. But not me. I marched into the ER full of rage and left a trail of verbal destruction in my wake. I got in trouble of course. The ER doc threatened to write me up, and my supervisor let me hear about it later, but I couldn't have cared less.

I learned a valuable lesson that night—I must put on the full armor of God *every* time I go to work, in fact, every time I leave my house. For I can't make it in this world without God's protection. And neither can you. You must put on the full armor of God too. Be strong in the Lord. Take up your shield and your sword and be strong in His mighty power.

PRAYER

Protect me from the enemy. Remind me to put on your full armor every day. Forgive me when I fail, Lord, and help me to be a gentleman regardless of what life throws my way.

APPLICATION

I was not prepared for that shift. My enemy, the devil, was lurking, using every opportunity to attack and slowly break me down, and he used another person to do it. She pushed me too far and I lost my cool. Describe a time you felt the same way. How did you react?

Read Ephesians 6:10-13. Why is it important for the Christian to put on the full armor of God every day? Who or what is it that we struggle against in life?

Reread verse 13. What will you be able to do once you have put on the full armor of God?

Answering the Call

Now read Ephesians 6:14-17. List the six different pieces of spiritual armor that are vital for the successful Christian walk.

God provided everything you need to stand your ground against your enemy. Are you wearing His full armor everyday? What practical steps might you now take to strengthen your daily walk with Christ?

BUILDING BLOCKS OF FAITH

The full armor of God—the belt of truth, the breastplate of righteousness, the helmet of salvation, the shield of faith, the sword of the spirit, and the gospel of Jesus Christ.

_____

_____

_____

_____

_____

_____

_____

_____

_____

_____

_____

_____

_____

_____

_____

_____

_____

_____

_____

Couldn't Do It Without You

Just as each of us has one body with many members,
and these members do not all have the same function,
so in Christ we who are many form one body, and
each member belongs to all the others. We have different gifts, according to the grace given us.
Romans 12:4-6

We first responders have it rough. We jump when others call, wallow in their blood, manage life-threatening emergencies and occasionally save lives. I'm proud to serve on the front lines of life, but my pride has its limits. I depend on other people. I could never do this job by myself. No way!

"Pat," Captain David Young shouted as I climbed from the ambulance. "You need to intubate him, dude. He's crashing fast!"

I grabbed my trauma bag and started toward the wreck. It looked bad, a Ford pickup wrapped around a tree, its front end crumpled in upon itself like aluminum foil. A team of firefighters and first responders scurried about the scene. Young knelt in the bed of the truck holding a bandage to the victim's head.

"Bring your suction unit too," he yelled. "He's full of blood!"

I ran back, grabbed the necessary equipment, and then trotted to the scene.

"It ain't good," Young said as I approached. "He was leaning against the tailgate when they hit the tree. Flew into the back of the cab headfirst." Young pulled away the trauma dressing. Blood poured from a gash in the center of the victim's head. He quickly recovered the wound and applied direct pressure. "Like I said, not good."

I gazed at my patient. His eyes looked lifeless. He breathed in short gurgling gasps. Young forced open his jaw. I inserted a hard plastic catheter.

"Okay," I said. "Turn it on."

My partner hit the power switch on the suction unit. A long line of bright red blood coursed up the tube. The catheter sucked and hissed, but I was unable to keep up with the steady stream of blood flowing into his mouth. I felt myself begin to panic.

"We're losing him," I said. "Help me!"

"Tell us what to do," somebody said.

"You two," I said pointing at two of the firefighters. "Get

a trauma line set up in the back of the truck. And one of you grab the backboard and stretcher." I handed my partner the catheter. "Here, you suction. I'll intubate."

The church is like that group of rescue workers, a team of believers, each with a different role. We all work together for one common good—to serve the Lord. To save people's lives.

And so, we did our jobs. My partner, the firefighters, the police officers controlling the crowd. We worked as a professional team. We suctioned. We intubated. We dressed the bleeding head wound and immobilized our patient. Then we drove him to the emergency room and left him in the doctors' care. We did everything within our collective power to achieve the impossible, to sustain our patient's life, but in my heart I knew he was already gone.

Are you a member of a Church? A group of believers who worship together and pray, each using the gifts he was given to serve the others and to spread the Gospel of the Lord Jesus Christ?

A few years later I transported a young woman to the hospital. She spoke of a bad wreck, of how a pickup truck had slammed into a tree. She'd been driving that evening. Her cousin had been the passenger, leaning against the tailgate when the accident occurred.

"He almost died," she explained. "The impact threw him forward. He hit his head on the cab. He lives on Holloway Street now. He's—"

Answering the Call

"Wait a minute," I said interrupting her. "What's your cousin's name?"

She told me.

I felt my eyes widen. "Are you telling me he's alive?"

"Oh, yes," she said. "His fingers still tingle a little, but otherwise he's fine. The paramedics saved him."

It wasn't just the paramedics who saved that man; it was David Young and the other firefighters, the police officers who helped us on the scene, the emergency department staff, the surgical team, and every other physician, nurse and physical therapist involved in his recovery. We worked together as a team, each member performing his or her role for the benefit of the victim, and together we accomplished the impossible.

Just like that special team, we in the church have been called to action. And you have a function. Are you performing it? Join a team of believers and start working for the Body of Christ today.

PRAYER

God, please bless all the men and women who work so tirelessly in the field of emergency response. They make a difference. They save lives. And sometimes, when we all work together, we can even accomplish the impossible.

Answering the Call

APPLICATION

Teamwork was vital to the success of that EMS call. All members worked together for the common good of the victim, and in the end we succeeded. He survived. Describe a situation where you responded as a member of a team.

What role did you play on the team?

Was the team successful? What would have happened if you had attempted to accomplish the same results alone?

What would have been the result if you had been missing from the team?

Read Romans 12:4-8. What does this passage have to say about the Body of Christ?

Answering the Call

What function are you providing in the Body of Christ? (Remember the Body is not complete unless every member is performing his/her role.)

BUILDING BLOCKS OF FAITH

One man's gift is to prophesy. Another's is to serve. One's is to encourage, and another's is to lead. One man's is to teach, and still another's is to show mercy.

Answering the Call

JOURNAL

_____

_____

_____

_____

_____

_____

_____

_____

_____

_____

_____

_____

_____

_____

_____

_____

_____

_____

_____

_____

Under His Mighty Wing

He that dwelleth in the secret place of the most
High shall abide under the shadow of the Almighty.
I will say of the LORD, He is my refuge and my for-
tress; my God; in Him I will trust.
Psalm 91:1-2

First Responders deal with potentially dangerous situations
every day. We go on emergency calls that demand a
heightened sense of awareness and a certain amount of
faith in our fellow man. I usually figure that, if I'm careful,
everything will be all right. But you and I know that life
is not always fair. Bad things do happen, even to good
people. So how should we prepare ourselves for the
dangerous moments in life? How can a person ever find
peace knowing that danger could lurk around every
corner?

My father once told me a story of a squadron of WWII
fighter pilots. The commander had his men memorize Psalm
91—a beautiful poem of God's promise of protection, His
angels, and the fortress He provides His people against
the perils of life. Every morning his men stood as a unit
and recited the passage before climbing into their planes

94

and flying off to fight the Germans. And as the story goes, not one of them was injured during the course of the war. Every man returned safely to his home.

The telling of that story by my father changed my life, for I now understand that God is my fortress. I take comfort in being by his side. Gain strength in knowing He is always there.

"Kim," I called to my wife. "Have you seen Dan?"

"No, I thought he was with you."

I sighed and walked through the house calling my son's name. I was used to it. Dan was a rascal. He was three years old, full of life, and we were late for church.

"Danny," I called. "Where are you, buddy?" Silence. I walked outside and called him again. Nothing. I trotted around the house shouting his name. Still no boy. "Dan?" I yelled. "Where are you?"

I sprinted back to the front of the house. "Kim. He's not here! I can't find him!"

My wife joined me in a frantic search. I felt confused. Desperate. Suddenly I heard a small voice. I ran to the side yard and saw my son walking from our neighbor's house. He had an apple in his hand and a huge smile on his face.

Answering the Call

I picked up my son and hugged him. I felt frustrated of course, and angry that he'd run off, but he was back home and safe and that was **all** that mattered. We talked about it. It was a short discussion, after all he was only a child, but later my father and I had a much longer chat.

"Son," my dad said, "listen to me. You won't always be there to watch over Dan. He's going to grow up, move out and have his own children, and someday, God forbid, no matter how much you pray for him, something bad **could** happen. That's life. You need to learn to trust the Lord."

That's when he told me the story of the squadron, and how we're to cling to the promises found in Psalm 91. "Do what those pilots did," he said. "Memorize that scripture, recite it every day, and then let Dan go. God will watch over him."

That was over twenty years ago and today Dan and his brother, Phillip, are healthy young men. God did watch over them, and now they are on their own. But, still, not a day goes by that I don't pray those precious words I memorized so long ago. Only now I can rest, for I know my boys are safe and sound, living in the shadow of God's mighty wing.

Do you live in fear? For your life or for that of a loved one? Cling to God's promises. He will help you tackle your fears. And He will walk with you and yours through the darkest valleys of life.

PRAYER

"Lord, hold my wife, my children, those I love in the palm of your hand. Give your angels charge over them today. Cover them with your feathers that under your mighty wings they might trust."

Answering the Call
APPLICATION

Everyone feels frightened from time to time. Describe a moment that you felt truly frightened, for a loved one, or for yourself.

What or whom did you cling to for strength?

Read Psalm 91. God promises a place where you may always find refuge. Where is it?

Who will He send to watch over you during times of need?

"Because he loves me," says the LORD, "I will rescue him." What else does God promise to do for you and your loved ones in this passage?

Would you memorize Psalm 91, and claim its promises every day for the rest of your life? If so, begin now by committing the first two verses to memory. Write the verses here and repeat them throughout the day until they have become engrained in your mind:

BUILDING BLOCKS OF FAITH

Like a mountain unmoved by the forces of time, The
Lord is my refuge. My rock. My salvation.

JOURNAL

_____

_____

_____

_____

_____

_____

_____

_____

_____

_____

_____

_____

_____

_____

_____

_____

_____

Created For Good Works

For we are God's workmanship, created in Christ Jesus
to do good works, which God prepared in advance for
us to do.
Ephesians 2:10

Thomas lived in a small group home on the south side
of town. He had AIDS, renal failure, high blood pressure,
and the night I met him an overall sick feeling he couldn't
explain. "I'm due for dialysis tomorrow," he said, "but
tonight I just don't feel right."

He didn't look right either. He was only 47, but he looked
old and tired as if he'd spent a lifetime on the run, fighting,
and struggling just to stay alive.

I wondered what had happened to him. Surely God had
created him for a reason, but had he lived a good life?
Done the best with what he had? Or had he chosen the
wrong path and ended up full of regret?

I performed a quick assessment. Checked his blood
pressure and pulse. I hooked up the cardiac monitor and
took a look at his heart. Physically he checked out okay,
but I sensed something deeper was wrong. I glanced at

his face and got the feeling that this was more than just a sick call. He needed to talk to someone. And I was okay with that. "Tell you what," I said. "Let's take a ride."

He smiled and rose to his feet. It was a routine transport. I stuck an 18-gauge IV catheter in his arm, took another look at his EKG, and then leaned back and looked at him as we rode down the highway.

"So, Thomas," I said. "Where are you from?"

"Right here."

"Yeah? Then you remember this place before it became a ghetto."

He nodded.

"Look," I said, "forgive me for prying, but, well, I was just wondering…were you ever in a gang?"

"A gang?" A stern expression tightened his face. "I learned to shoot a gun when I was five years old. Started taking drugs when I was twelve. Did heroin for more than twenty years on the street and then every day in prison for seven more. It won't my mom that taught me all that."

Have you made poor decisions? Feel that you've lost your way? It's not too late to turn around. Jesus is there to help you find your way back.

I gazed at Thomas without speaking. I felt he deserved that.

Answering the Call

"The alcohol and drugs ruined me. My kidneys are shot now. I don't blame nobody else though. I made the mistakes, and I'll live with 'em. But these gangs you asked about?" He paused and shook his head. "They're bad, man. These kids today will shoot anybody. They steal and rob for drugs. They kill. And those girls? They only keep 'em round for one reason—makin' babies. To the gangs that's all they're good for. My daughter's in one now, you know." He glanced at me as if searching for an answer. "She stays coked up and pregnant most the time."

"Can't you talk to her?" I asked. "Try to help her?"

"No, man, you don't get it. Can't never talk to her no more. Afraid of her. I know it's my fault, she's my child, but that one…she won't created for no good."

I felt a strange paradox as I walked away from the ER: pleased to know that Thomas is a Christian today—he gave his life to Christ somewhere along the way—but saddened by what I had just witnessed: Harsh reality. Not just words from some magazine article about gangs and troubled youth, but real flesh and blood, a grown man who survived the streets only to live and suffer the consequences of his mistakes.

If you've made serious mistakes and feel that you've lost your way, don't surrender. God created you for a reason, to live a good life and to do the best you can with what He gave you. Turn to Him. He loves you. He will help you find your way.

PRAYER

Lord, help me to remember that I am Your workmanship. Give me the strength to make sound decisions today, and to turn away from the path of sin that eventually leads to death.

Answering the Call

APPLICATION

Most likely you have lived what you believe to be a good life. Take a few moments to think about your life. Compose a list of your most important accomplishments.

Do you believe that any of these accomplishments will earn you the right to go to Heaven?

Read Ephesians 2:8-10. What does the scripture say regarding good works?

Why then is it important to live a good life? Read Matthew 5:16, 1 Peter 2:12. According to these verses, what is accomplished as a result of your good works?

Remember salvation is free, but we will all be judged according to the works that we do (See Psalm 9:7-8, and Ecclesiastes 12:13-14). How might this knowledge change your daily life? What steps will you take to glorify your Heavenly Father?

BUILDING BLOCKS OF FAITH

Doing good works saves no one, but all will be judged
for the works that they do.

JOURNAL

_____

_____

_____

_____

_____

_____

_____

_____

_____

_____

_____

_____

_____

_____

_____

Well, what did you expect?

*Love your enemies, do good to them, and lend
to them without expecting to get anything back.
Then your reward will be great, and you will be
sons of the Most High, because he is kind to the
ungrateful and wicked.*
Luke 6:35

Larry was a junkie. I think he had more toxic chemicals in his veins than blood. I found him lying in the bushes barely breathing, his eyes half-open, pupils like pinpoints. Foamy saliva dripped from the corner of his mouth. Track marks scarred both arms. I knelt beside him, pulled a dirty syringe from his arm, and then opened my med box to prepare a syringe of my own.

"What else do you want?" my partner, Warren, asked me.

"We need an IV."

"You know he's just gonna rip it out, don't you?"

Answering the Call

I glanced at Larry's face and remembered the last time we'd seen him. The way he'd cussed us out. Treated us with disdain. But then I remembered the scripture…love your enemies. Be kind to others even when you don't expect to receive anything in return.

"Probably," I said, "but let's do it anyway, Warren. Okay?"

"Suit yourself."

Warren shrugged and snatched a 500-cc IV bag from the med box. I wrapped a tourniquet around Larry's arm, thumped up a fat vein, and then jabbed an IV catheter deep into the vessel. The flash chamber filled with blood. I threaded the catheter and attached the IV tubing. Warren set the flow rate to keep the vein open.

Next I selected a small plastic vial and stuck a 3-cc syringe into the round rubbery top. I turned the bottle over, pulled back on the plunger and withdrew two milliliters of clear fluid. After tapping the syringe to clear it of excess air bubbles I attached it to the IV line and pushed the drug into Larry's vein.

Mere seconds passed before his eyes began to flutter. His respirations quickened. He slurped a couple of times as if sucking the remains of a milkshake from a straw and then took a deep breath and sat up. He looked sluggish at first, blurry and unseeing as if covered by a thick haze, but then his constricted pupils dilated and his mental status sharpened to a fine point.

"Hey," I said. "Welcome back."

Answering the Call

"What happened?"

"You OD'd again," Warren said. "You almost stopped breathing this time, Larry."

I offered Larry my hand to help him up. He slapped it away. "You took away my high, man!" He ripped the IV out of his arm and gave me the finger. Then he stormed off, bleeding from the punctured vein and shouting obscenities at us as he stumbled down the street. I felt stunned. I glanced at my partner.

"Did you see that?"

"Well, what'd you expect?" Warren said. "A thank you note?"

Later I thought about what had happened, about my own highs and lows, and about the many times I've slapped God's hand away when He was trying to help me up. Am I any different than Larry? Are you? You know we all crave the high of lustful living, but in the end that path leads to addiction and death. Christ came to save us from ourselves, to turn us away from the sin that entangles us. So the next time you feel convicted by the helpful words of a friend, don't turn them away. Christ may have sent them to lend you a helping hand.

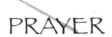

PRAYER

Lord, forgive me for the times I may have cursed you, spit in your face, or blamed you for my mistakes. Help me to forgive others when they do the same to me.

Answering the Call

APPLICATION

Have you ever been blamed for someone else's mistake? Or rejected or rebuked when you were only trying to help? How did it make you feel? Describe your feelings.

Read John 19:1-18. What does this passage tell us that Pilate and the Roman soldiers did to Jesus Christ?

Read Isaiah 53:5-6 and 1 Peter 2:24-25. Why was it necessary for Christ to suffer this brutal punishment?

Now read Luke 23:34. What did Christ ask the Father to do as He hung upon the cross? Was He speaking only of those present at the time, or was He also speaking of you?

Christ suffered and died so that you might live. He paid the ultimate sacrifice for you. Will you respond differently the next time you are ridiculed, rejected, or unjustly blamed for another's mistake?

BUILDING BLOCKS OF FAITH

Anyone can love someone back, but to love one's enemies—those who persecute you and revile you and speak harshly about you behind your back—that is the mark of a true Christian.

JOURNAL

_____

_____

_____

_____

_____

_____

_____

_____

_____

_____

_____

_____

_____

What's your gift?

Each one should use whatever gift he has received
to serve others, faithfully administering God's
grace in its various forms.
1 Peter 4:10

"How're you doing, brother? Working hard or hardly working?"

My friend, Steve, always greets me that way. It's his trademark and I love it. It usually makes me laugh, helps me prepare for the shift. But I didn't feel much like laughing that night. My heart was heavy. I needed to talk. Steve clocked in and followed me out to the ambulance bay to check the truck.

"So," he said opening the airway bag. "What's bothering you, brother?"

Steve may not have realized it, but at that moment he was doing what the scripture tells us to do, administering God's grace to me. Using his gift of friendship to admonish and build me up. And boy, did I need it.

I shrugged. "I didn't realize it showed."

Answering the Call

"It shows." Steve gave the wrench atop the oxygen bottle a twist. He glanced at the regulator, nodded, and then retightened it and slid the cylinder back into the bag. "You wanna talk?"

"You know that book I've been writing? It was rejected again."

"No way."

"Another publisher said no. But that's not all. This time my agent sent the manuscript back to me. She's giving up on it. Says she can't sell it."

"Hmmm." Steve bit his lip as if trying to hold back a smile. "I probably shouldn't tell you this," he said with a grin, "but deep down, I'm kind of glad."

"Glad?"

"Well, ever since you started writing that book your head's been somewhere else. Your heart's not here anymore, dude. It's like you've already left."

"Steve, I've been writing for over five years. I've worked hard to get published. You don't know how—"

"You've worked hard for this!"

"This? Steve, this job's chewed me up and spit me out so many times I can't think straight anymore. I mean, c'mon, man. We work all the time. We wallow in blood and guts. We go places most people wouldn't get close to. And where's the payoff? When am I ever going to get mine?"

"Is that why you write? To get yours?"

Steve's question hit a raw nerve. It hurt me, because deep inside I knew he was right. God has blessed me so much. How selfish of me to take one of His gifts and use it for personal gain. Are you doing that too? Seeking recognition? Money? Personal pleasure or fame?

"Well," I said with an awkward stammer, "that's not the only reason."

"Look, you may not want to hear this, brother, but I believe God put you here for a reason, and it's not to make money. He's using you in more ways than you know. I mean just think of all the lives you've touched. The people you've saved over the last twenty years. All those students you've trained to be great paramedics. Brother, there are a lot of folks out there who would be much worse off today if not for you. Shoot, a lot of 'em wouldn't even be here."

"So, what am I supposed to do? Just give it all up?"

"No, write. But do it for the right reason. And don't even think about giving up EMS. God's given you a wonderful gift, brother. You need to *use it!*"

If you're using God's gifts for the wrong reasons then it's time you made a change too. Discover your gifts, then get out there and use them for the right reason—to serve the Lord.

PRAYER

Heavenly Father, please forgive me for being so selfish. And thank you for my good friend, Steve. For using him to remind me how truly blessed I am. I'm a paramedic, set apart to save lives. That is my calling. That is my gift.

Answering the Call

APPLICATION

Do you have talents or abilities that set you apart from others? Take a few moments now to create a short list. What are you "good at"?

Read Romans 12:6-8. According to the scripture, how did you acquire these abilities or talents?

Now read Ecclesiastes 9:10. How does God expect you to use these gifts?

Colossians 3:23. For whose glory are you to use your gifts?

According to Galatians 5:19 selfish ambition is just as much a sin as idolatry, drunkenness and sexual immorality. Are you selfishly using the gifts God gave you for your own edification, or are you using them to serve Him?

BUILDING BLOCKS OF FAITH

There are many kinds of gifts, but there is only one Holy Spirit who freely gives them. A gift is something God expects you to use for His glory. For the edification of the church.

JOURNAL

Are you ready for this?

Nothing in all creation is hidden from God's sight.
Everything is uncovered and laid bare before the
eyes of him to whom we must give account.
Hebrew 4:13-14

I had just finished writing an EMS report at the hospital when a fellow paramedic shouted at me from the other side of the emergency room. "Pat," he said urgency on his face. "Get over here quick. You need to see this!"

"What is it?"

"Car wreck. Hurry."

I put aside my paperwork and walked across the ER into Trauma Room-1. A large crowd stood around the gurney. I didn't find that unusual. That particular ER belongs to a teaching hospital, so it's quite common to find people standing around watching the doctors work—stabilizing critical patients, sewing up flesh, replacing precious blood. But as we pushed into the room, I sensed something wrong. The crowd seemed hungry instead of curious, wide-eyed and full of glee. Their lustful expressions seemed completely out of place.

Answering the Call

"What's going on?" I asked.

"Are you ready for this?" My co-worker pushed me to the center of the room. "Look."

My eyes flew open wide. A teenaged girl lay on the gurney stripped of all clothing, her figure laid bare for everyone in the room to see. She was about eighteen years old with beautiful blue eyes and long blonde hair. She had a goose egg on the right side of her head. A trace amount of blood stained her cheek and nose. But otherwise she looked unscathed, the victim of a traffic accident that had apparently knocked her out.

I felt stunned. The physicians and nurses were justified in being there, of course. They were the trauma team, they had a job to do. And the removal of clothing is an essential component of the major trauma assessment. Everything must be uncovered to allow for critical judgment of the injuries at hand. But the onlookers? I saw no reason for the rest of the crowd. A dozen men stood there gawking. The poor girl was being violated.

I felt ashamed. I walked out of the room.

I never learned the extent of her injuries, but God used that young woman to teach me a valuable lesson. One day we will all be uncovered, our hearts laid bare before God. And no deed, no thought, no ill-conceived fantasy or spoken word will remain hidden from His view. We will be exposed exactly as we are.

Answering the Call

Will you be ready when the King of Kings appears? When the Lord God exposes your sins and judges you for all you have done? If you know Jesus Christ you have nothing to fear. His blood covers you, washes you white as snow. But if you don't know Him, eternal judgment awaits, and after that—death. So turn your life over to Jesus Christ today. He is coming back, and when He does there will be no place on Earth to hide.

PRAYER

"Heavenly Father, I am a sinner. Thank you for sacrificing your Son for me. His shed blood covers my sins. And on the Day of Judgment, as I kneel before your throne, you won't see my filthiness at all. You will see his blood instead."

APPLICATION

Do you have any secrets? Things that you would prefer no one else ever knew? Well God knows. Psalm 33:15 says He considers everything you do. Read Proverbs 5:21…what does this passage say regarding your actions, your attitudes, your innermost secrets?

Now read Jeremiah 32:17-19. How will God reward you?

Also read Hebrews 4:12-14. List four attributes of God's word and the relevance of these in regard to your secret life.

According to this passage, what aspect of your life is hidden from God's view?

Are you a Christian? Are you living a life of obedience or are you ignoring His commands. Remember, nothing you do, say, or even think is hidden from God.

BUILDING BLOCKS OF FAITH

God's word penetrates. It divides. It judges the thoughts
and attitudes of the heart.

JOURNAL

_____

_____

_____

_____

_____

_____

_____

_____

_____

_____

_____

_____

_____

_____

_____

God Still Knows Exactly What To Do

So do not fear, for I am with you; do not be dismayed, for I am your God. I will strengthen you and help you; I will uphold you with my righteous right hand.
Isaiah 41:10

"I don't know what to do!"

Actress Jennifer Garner spoke that line in the 2001 Academy Award winning film, Pearl Harbor. She starred as Sandra, a young Army nurse serving in a makeshift hospital on Pearl Harbor on the morning of December 7, 1941. Walking wounded arrived by the score, bleeding profusely, their charred and broken bodies beaten to shreds, many with wounds too deep to fix. The doctors, nurses and Army corpsmen did everything they could to manage the unfathomable catastrophe, but the scene was overwhelming. It was too much to manage, too unbelievable to comprehend. Terrified, the young nurse looked around her at the mayhem and cried, "I don't know what to do!"

Answering the Call

Have you ever been so frightened you didn't know what to do? Well God has the answer. And He promised to provide you strength in those moments, to pick you up and carry you through the darkest hours of your life.

I can only imagine the horrors of that infamous day when our nation came under attack. Bombs fell from the sky. Torpedoes exploded. Over 2,300 brave sailors died and countless more were injured. It was the first time in modern history that we felt the pounding of our enemy's feet on our own soil—this sacred ground, the United States of America—and it angered us! We knew our enemy. We saw the whites of his eyes and the evil of his cause, and in our righteous determination we fought back. And thank God, we won!

But 70 years later we live in a different America. Our moral values have slipped. We've grown politically correct. And the godly principles on which this country was founded no longer seem important. Have we forgotten all that God has done for us?

Well make no mistake—we need Him again. Our world is at war, and just as in 1941 we are the battleground. Only this time we can't see our enemy. We don't know whom to trust. And many Americans have floundered, looking around them at the chaos and crying, "I don't know what to do!"

Well this is still sacred ground. America is still worth fighting for. And God is still in control. So stand up. Remember the Christian principles on which our country was founded. Turn to the one in whom we still trust. And stand your ground. God said, *"Do not fear, for I am with you; do not be dismayed, for I am your God. I will strengthen you and help you; I will uphold you with my righteous right hand."*

So I ask you, as you consider the fate of our great nation—this indivisible union that still provides liberty and justice for all—what are you so worried about? Why are you so afraid? God is still in charge. And if we will humble ourselves, turn back to Him and ask Him to heal our land, in His righteous determination He will do just that. He's still in charge. And He still knows exactly what to do.

PRAYER

"God, strengthen us now during this most crucial hour. Help us. Hold us in your hand and restore in us the principles that once made this nation great. You are God. You know exactly what to do."

APPLICATION

Has there ever been a time when you had absolutely no idea what to do? Take a moment and describe the circumstances.

How did you feel at the time? Scared? Confused?

Read Joshua 1:1-9. What encouragement did God give the Israelites three times in this passage?

What promise does this passage provide regarding God's presence in your life?

BUILDING BLOCKS OF FAITH

If God's people, who are called by His name, will humble themselves, pray, seek His face and turn from their wicked ways, then He will hear from heaven, forgive their sins, and heal their land.

Answering the Call

JOURNAL

_____

_____

_____

_____

_____

_____

_____

_____

_____

_____

_____

_____

_____

_____

_____

_____

_____

The Best of the Best

Whatever your hand finds to do, do it with all your might.
Ecclesiastes 9:10

To be the **best**: To excel, to outdo all others, to reach a level of accomplishment unsurpassed in one's field. And for a brave young man I know—my good friend's son— it means even more than that. It means to be willing to lay down his life, to sacrifice his freedom that others might live.

"Pat-Man, I need your help. They've called him up again. They're sending my son back over there. I called to ask for your prayers."

As my friend explained the situation I could hear the fear in his voice. I assured him I would pray for his son, and that everything would be all right, but my heart felt heavy as I hung up the phone. His young man had just gotten home, retired from the military and started a bright new career as a firefighter and EMT, and suddenly, without warning, they had decided to call him back. It didn't seem right. Why couldn't they just leave him alone?

Answering the Call

But deep inside I knew the reason why. It's because he's one of the best shooters in the U.S. Army. One of the elite. The best of the best.

Has God given you a special talent? A unique ability? A particular skill He wants you to use?

I've known many brave 1st responders: police officers and firefighters, EMTs and paramedics. Men and women with tough jobs who work hard to save other lives. But this young soldier has the hardest job of all. Surgical removal. One shot, one kill.

"A sniper! Hey, wait a minute. Pulling a trigger and deliberately killing another man? How can that be right?"

Well the Bible is full of similar stories. Men who were called on to fight, to play a part in God's divine plan. Take King David for instance, a man after God's own heart. As a young boy he attacked and killed the giant Philistine with a sling and a single stone. God called Him to battle and gave him the strength to complete the task. And Samson, a man made strong by God's own hand. The Spirit of the Lord came upon him in power, and he killed a thousand Philistines with the jawbone of a donkey.

Sometimes God uses rough men to accomplish His will. Men who are willing to use the gifts He gave them, to follow orders regardless of the cost. So when I consider this young man's sacrifices, his skills and his God-given talents, I suddenly understand what it means to be the best. It means to do whatsoever your hand finds to do, and to do it with all of your might.

Answering the Call

Are you doing the best you can with the gifts and talents God gave you? Don't waste another day. Find out what it is God has called you to do, and then do it. He will give you the power you need to succeed.

PRAYER

"Lord, please tell him how proud I am to know him, how much his sacrifice means, and how much I appreciate his willingness to fight…for my family, for my country, for my home. Honor and bless him, Lord. Grant him the strength to do his job well, and then bring him back home again so that he, too, may enjoy the blessings of liberty for which he has fought."

APPLICATION

Write a list of the jobs you have had in your life, or some of the important tasks you have been asked to accomplish. Afterwards, read each one aloud and ask yourself the following question—did I do my best?

Read the scripture passage again. What are you commanded to do when you work, whatever the task?

Now read Colossians 3:22-24. When you work, whom do you serve?

And why is it important to work at your job with all of your heart?

BUILDING BLOCKS OF FAITH

Make wise decisions. Use your time wisely. In the grave where you are going there is no more work. No more planning. No more wisdom. No more knowledge.

JOURNAL

_____

_____

_____

_____

_____

_____

_____

_____

_____

_____

_____

_____

_____

_____

_____

_____

_____

_____

_____

_____

Rejoice! It's Christmas!

For the wages of sin is death, but the gift of God is
eternal life in Christ Jesus our Lord.
Romans 6:23

Oh, Lord, not now. It's Christmas…

Larry's compressions were perfect. Two inches deep, a
hundred a minute, right out of the book. John had the
airway under control, an endotracheal tube in place,
properly secured and ventilated. My partner, A.J., started
the IV and handed me drugs. Epinephrine. Atropine.
I pushed them into the IV line, delivering just the right
amount to stimulate the old man's heart. In all it was a
perfectly run code, an organized attempt to save a human
life. It could not have gone any better. But deep inside I
knew it was futile, he wasn't going to make it.

"I don't know," I said shaking my head. "This just isn't
working. I think it's time to stop." I glanced at A.J. "What
do you think?"

"No," a voice behind me said. "Please don't stop! C'mon,
daddy," the young woman cried. "You can do it!"

136

Answering the Call

I glanced around me at my patient's family, a wife and three grown children. Their cries of support, the hope I saw on their faces, it all just about broke my heart. We'd done everything right, run a perfect code in the middle of their living room—a beautiful home decorated with Christmas tree and lights—but a flat green line traced across the ECG screen. It painted a picture of finality, a portrait of hopelessness and death.

"It's Christmas, dad. You can't leave us now!"

"Honey, stay with us," his wife cried. "We need you here."

If there were no sin in the world, there would be no death. But we live in an imperfect world. Everyone sins. We all fall short of God's standard. Therefore death is inevitable. But, oh Lord, sometimes it hurts so much…

I felt my eyes well up. I shook my head. "It's no use. He's already had three rounds of epi and atropine. One of bicarb. Pacemaker won't capture…"

I paused and glanced at the family again. I could feel their pain, sense their loss. But as I considered my protocol I knew what I had to do.

"Larry," I said my heart breaking as I spoke the words, "hold compressions."

I placed my fingertips against the old man's neck. Larry took a much-needed breather. I squinted and stared at the cardiac monitor hoping to detect a sign of life—a blip, a pulse, any indication that my patient's heart had responded to treatment—but the thin green line continued its lonely trek across the screen. My fingers felt nothing but cool dry skin beneath them. No pulse. No warmth. No life.

I glanced at Larry and shook my head.

"You can stop."

I stood and faced the family.

"Folks…"

I took a deep breath. A fist-sized lump threatened to close my throat.

"I'm so sorry."

It's hard to lose a loved one, especially when our thoughts turn homeward and old memories of Christmas fill us with hope and joy, but there's never a convenient time. Death always seems to surprise us. It's so final, and at times seems so unfair. So what's a family to do when they face such terrible loss? Where can they find peace? Where's the hope?

In Christ alone.

If we were totally obedient to God we wouldn't need a savior. But we're not. The Bible says we have all sinned. And with sin comes eternal darkness. But let the world rejoice, for two thousand years ago God sent his son, Jesus Christ, our one and only promise for everlasting life.

PRAYER

"I was destined to die but you saved me. Thank
you for Christmas, for a new beginning, for
everlasting life."

APPLICATION

Are you totally obedient to God? Of course not. No one is perfect. James 3:2 reads, "**We all stumble in many ways**." Read Romans 3:23. What does the Bible say we all have in common?

In what areas of your life do you feel that you are being disobedient to God?

Now read Romans 6:23. What will happen to each of us as a result of this failure?

What is God's solution to this problem?

God has offered you the free gift of eternal life? Have you accepted it? If not will you do so today? If you have accepted Christ will you decide today to live a life of obedience? What steps will you now take toward that commitment?

140

Answering the Call

BUILDING BLOCKS OF FAITH

Jesus Christ: Wonderful Counselor, Mighty God,
Everlasting Father, Prince of Peace.

JOURNAL

_____

_____

_____

_____

_____

_____

_____

_____

_____

_____

_____

_____

_____

_____

_____

_____

We Need a Revival!

"For God so loved the world that he gave his one and only Son, that whoever believes in him shall not perish but have eternal life."
John 3:16

Someone needs to tell these kids. They're all gonna die if they keep living like this…

"Medic-7," the station loudspeaker announced. "Got one shot!"

I grabbed my stethoscope and followed my partner to the ambulance wondering what we would find when we arrived on scene this time. Another gang member? Another kid? I had learned to expect almost anything. Our streets had become a ghetto. A cesspool of drugs and crime.

"A teenaged male shot once in the head," the dispatcher continued. "Police officer on the scene requesting Code-3 response. Code-3."

"10-4," my partner responded jumping behind the wheel and keying the mike. "Medic-7 en route."

Answering the Call

I climbed into the passenger seat and buckled up. I grabbed a pair of latex gloves and pulled one on each hand as my partner pulled into traffic. I tried to calm myself as he hurried to the scene. *Relax. You've been a medic for a long time. You've seen this before.* But as we pulled onto Hopkins Street I felt my stomach tighten. My palms began to sweat. There's just something unsettling about a young man with a bullet hole in the side of his head, his life blood spilling out all over the ground and a dangerous crowd pressing in on you demanding you get to work.

There was nothing we could do of course. But for the sake of our own skins and the fact that we were standing on their turf and outnumbered about a hundred to one, we made a good show of it. We loaded him up and moved to the truck assuring the angry crowd we would do our best to save him. Once clear of the scene, however, my partner killed the lights and sirens and slowed down to normal traffic. I stared into the victim's lifeless eyes trying to guess his age. Eighteen years old, maybe? Nineteen? Oh, Lord, what a waste.

"Duke ER," I said keying the radio mike. "I'm sorry but we're bringing you a corpse. Another gang member got shot. There's nothing we can do."

For that young man, no, there was nothing we could do. But it's not too late to help the others, the kids still out there on our streets. It's time for a revival. Time to take Christ's message of hope to the broken world of our inner cities.

Answering the Call

Have you witnessed the hopelessness in our society? The violence and pain? Are you doing anything about it?

Let's take our streets captive for Jesus. Take the gospel out there and see what God can do. For God so loved the world that He gave His only son, for these young people, and indeed, for the entire world.

PRAYER

"Help us retake our city for Christ. I ask for power and protection, for the First Responders who are out there everyday sharing the love of Christ. Give us opportunities to reach those who have no hope, and the courage to risk it all for the Lord. Dear God, we need a revival.

Answering the Call

APPLICATION

Our streets are full of people who need to hear the Gospel. But then so are our schools, our neighborhoods, the places we all go to work. Did any person come to mind when you read this devotion? Write down their name.

Describe them—what do they look like? What color are their eyes?

What is it about that person that draws you to them?

Read John 3:16 again. For whom did God send His only son?

Would you be so bold as to pray for this person, and then to go to them to tell them about Jesus Christ? What steps will you now take?

BUILDING BLOCKS OF FAITH

God's promise is for you, and for your children, for all who are
far off, even as many as the Lord our God shall call.

JOURNAL

Coolest of the Cool

Boldly and without hindrance he preached the kingdom of God and taught about the Lord Jesus Christ.

Acts 28:31

I couldn't believe it! He was the coolest of the cool, onetime warlord of the most vicious gang that had ever roamed the streets of New York City, and he was coming to town. I had to see him!

I'd read his book. Well, at least part of it. I couldn't get enough of the rumbles, the switchblades, and the blood, but when he started talking about God, I put the book down. I just wasn't interested in hearing about salvation. But what I didn't realize at thirteen years of age was that God *was* interested in me. He had a plan for my life, and it began the day I picked up that book—***Run Baby, Run***.

"Nicky Cruz? He's coming to town?"

Wild with anticipation I put on my denim jacket and boots. I slid a fake switchblade into my pocket and followed my sister downtown. The auditorium was packed. A feeling of intensity gripped the room. And then I saw him step

148

to the podium. I gazed in amazement. He was everything I had imagined and more. Solid. Tough looking and scarred. I couldn't believe I was actually looking at Nicky Cruz.

He spoke of the ghetto, and of zip guns and chains and blood. And the excitement I'd felt when I'd first read his book hit me all over again. But as he shared the rest of his story I felt a deep yearning. Whatever that tough Puerto Rican kid had found after years of fighting and running from God—I wanted it.

"Jesus saved me," Nicky exclaimed, "and he can save you too!"

The service drew to a close. Nicky gave the altar call. I inched forward with a hundred other people. I didn't even know why. But then Nicky prayed and something remarkable happened to me, and since that moment my life has never been the same.

"Did you do it?" my sister asked me at the conclusion of the service. "Did you pray?"

"Nah," I said, coolly shaking my head. "I just wanted to see what he looked like. He was cool!"

But I did do it—I bowed my head that night and prayed to receive Christ. So thank you, Nicky. God used you to ignite a fire in me. I thank God for your boldness. I thank God for you. You are still my hero. The coolest of the cool!

Answering the Call

Have you met the Lord Jesus? Have you responded to his call? If not, don't waste another day. Get down on your knees right now and invite Christ into your life. Take it from a man who knows—from a naïve teenaged boy who responded almost forty years ago—you'll be glad you did.

PRAYER

"Thank you, Heavenly Father, for sending Nicky Cruz. Now send me. There are others who need to know. And fill me with that same boldness, Lord. For if Jesus can save Nicky and me, then He can save them too."

Answering the Call

APPLICATION

If not for a brave young preacher named David Wilkerson, Nicky Cruz may have never heard about the Lord Jesus Christ. And if not for Nicky, I may have never heard. What about you? Who first told you about Christ? Have you made a decision to follow Him? If not will you do so now?

If you have already given your life to Christ, have you shared your faith with anyone else? Read Hebrews 13:16. Why is it important to share your faith with others?

Read Acts 4:1-20. How did Peter and John respond (v. 20) when ordered by the rulers and elders to stop speaking of or teaching about the Lord Jesus?

Do you share their zeal? If not do you feel that you should?

How different might your life be today if no one had bothered to tell you about Christ? Will you commit to sharing the Gospel of Jesus Christ with someone you know?

BUILDING BLOCKS OF FAITH

Remember it only takes one spark to ignite a raging fire.

JOURNAL

_____

_____

_____

_____

_____

_____

_____

_____

_____

_____

_____

_____

_____

_____

_____

_____

A Child is Born

For unto us a child is born, unto us a son is given;
and the government shall be on his shoulder; and
his name shall be called Wonderful, Counselor, The
mighty God, The everlasting Father,
The Prince of Peace.
Isaiah 9:6 (KJV)

"Hey, I know you!"

I stared at the woman trying to make a connection. She looked vaguely familiar to me, standing in the booking area of the police station with handcuffs about her wrists, but I couldn't place her face.

"You delivered my baby," she said as the arresting officer removed the cuffs. "Six months ago in the elevator? Remember?"

And suddenly I did remember. Oh, how I remembered…

The house was cluttered. Dingy and hot. A drunk, heavyset male lay passed out on the living room floor.

Answering the Call

She lay by his side in the middle of the room cursing, her knees apart, her swollen belly exposed. "How far along are you?" I asked kneeling to begin my assessment.

"Don't touch me," she shouted. "Take me to the hospital!"

"Relax, I'm going to help you."

"I don't want your help. I want a ride!"

Her face drew up tight. She took a breath and held it. Her cheeks turned red. And then suddenly a loud cry burst forth. She moaned and screamed and panted and cried until the contraction eased. Then she sat there panting, angry and belligerent. And the rest of the call was pretty much the same. She griped and complained all the way to the hospital, fussing about her treatment in life and all of the bad things people had done to her. "They don't understand. I deserve better." And on, and on, and on.

I ignored her vulgar language and pulled together the equipment for a complicated delivery, all the time praying for the baby yet to be born. We backed into the ambulance bay. My partner opened the doors. We wheeled her inside the hospital and entered the elevator that would take us upstairs to Labor & Delivery. Another contraction gripped her. "It's coming," she screamed as the elevator began to rise. "Oh God, it's out!"

I lifted the sheet that covered her and saw a small baby boy lying on the stretcher between her legs—small and blue and slippery looking. And still.

Answering the Call

I picked him up and quickly toweled him off. Then I suctioned his mouth and nose. I vigorously rubbed his tiny back to stimulate respiration. Finally he gasped and took a shallow breath. I rushed him into Labor & Delivery with my partner pushing the stretcher at my heels. The nurses welcomed us warmly, but as they realized the baby's distressed condition they quickly took over and went to work.

I felt the excitement one can only understand upon having witnessed the arrival of a new life, but my heart could not rejoice. I didn't know if he would survive. And a few moments later, when the doctor told me the mother had confessed to smoking crack that night, I became almost sick. "That poor child," I murmured. "He doesn't have a chance."

He did live, but upon seeing his mother in the booking area of the police department I realized all over again that the poor child had a tough life ahead. I still pray that he makes it.

When I think of this child's birth and the circumstances surrounding his untimely delivery, I am reminded of another poor baby born in a lonely stable in Bethlehem, before hospitals, before medical care. Who would have thought *he* had a chance? But he came. He lived. He died on a cross and rose from the dead to bring hope to a dying world. Without Christ none of us have a chance. But be of good cheer, it's Christmas, and unto you a savior was born—Jesus Christ the Lord.

PRAYER

Heavenly Father, protect that baby boy. Make him healthy and strong. And one day, when the time is just right, have someone tell him about Jesus. The Everlasting Father. Prince of Peace.

APPLICATION

Two thousand years ago a baby was born under the worst of conditions. He spent his first night in a crib made of wood and lined with animal fodder. Read the scripture again, Isaiah 9:6…what are some of the names given to that baby boy?

Now continue by reading the next verse, Isaiah 9:7. What does this passage indicate that he will accomplish?

Many people are born under bad conditions. Others live their entire lives struggling simply to survive. But it is never hopeless, for unto us a child was born. Unto us a savior was given. How might this knowledge change the way you think about your current situation? About another person you know?

BUILDING BLOCKS OF FAITH
Jesus loves the little children, all the little children of the world.

Answering the Call

JOURNAL

_____

_____

_____

_____

_____

_____

_____

_____

_____

_____

_____

_____

_____

_____

_____

_____

_____

_____

_____

_____

Do You Believe This?

Jesus said, "I am the resurrection and the life. He
who believes in me will live, even though he dies;
and whoever lives and believes in me will never die.
Do you believe this?"
John 11:25-26

We call it a Code. Someone else's heart has stopped
beating, and our response—how well we manage
our crews and our skills and our abilities to hold it all
together—can determine whether the victim lives or dies.
It's a scenario paramedics and EMT's practice over and
over again to perfection. A rapid response followed by a
few moments of controlled fury as we feverishly struggle
to save another person's life. And sometimes our practice
pays off. This time, however, there was nothing my partner
and I could do…

"Medic-seven," the dispatcher said, her voice echoing
across the ambulance bay. "Cardiac arrest."

My heart skipped a beat.

"A ninety-two year old female," the dispatcher continued.
"Not breathing."

Answering the Call

My partner entered the address into the GPS unit. I hit the gas. We made excellent time weaving through traffic and arrived on scene only four minutes after the dispatch, but it wasn't soon enough. Our patient was already gone. She lay on the floor beside her bed with no sign of life. Her eyes, frosty and opaque, painted a picture of recent death. Her heart was silent. It was easy to see she was gone.

The Bible says that those who believe in Christ will **never** die. That if you call on His name you will live forever. Do you believe this?

I felt sad as we drove back to the station. Another life had ended, and there was nothing I could do about it. I backed the truck into the bay and was just about to climb out of it when we received another call. Another cardiac arrest. Only this time the victim was much younger, only four months old. We found her lying in bed, her tiny limbs stiff and cool, her skin a sickening shade of blue.

I felt my heart break. I glanced at the young family standing on the other side of the room. I wanted to say something to them but couldn't find the words. On the children's faces I saw shocked innocence, on their mother's unimaginable pain. A bright Christmas tree glowed in the corner of the room but it seemed to lack the luster it might have just hours earlier, before death entered their home robbing them of Christmas joy.

Answering the Call

Have you ever lost a loved one unexpectedly? Felt the sting of death? The realization that there was nothing you could have done to prevent it?

The loss of these two fragile lives should serve as a grim reminder that death is inevitable. No man knows when his time will come. As fish are caught in a cruel net, or birds are caught in a snare, we all fall victim to physical death sooner or later. So consider this: Jesus said, "I am the resurrection and the life. He who believes in me will never die." Physical death will happen, it's true, but the spirit can live on forever. Do you believe this?

Ask Jesus Christ to be your Savior and Lord. Do it today. And if you already know Him introduce Him to someone you love, for no man knows when his hour will come.

PRAYER

"Heavenly Father, when I witness death I can't help but wonder—did that person know you? Did they accept your gift of everlasting life? Give me the courage to tell another person, Lord. There are so many people who still don't know."

APPLICATION

Have you ever lost a loved one? Do you find yourself wondering where they will spend eternity? The scriptures are clear on this matter. Read John 3:1-7. What does Christ say here regarding the Kingdom of Heaven?

Now read John 1:1-14. Who is "the Word" that John was referring to in verse 1 where he wrote, "In the beginning was the Word, and the Word was with God, and the Word was God"?

Do you believe this? That Christ was here from the beginning and is in fact, God?

Take a look at 1John 1:9. What must a man do to be born again?

There are many people in your life that do not know where they will spend eternity. Read Matthew 28:16-20. What is your responsibility as a follower of Jesus Christ?

BUILDING BLOCKS OF FAITH
Live for today, it may be your last day on earth.

JOURNAL

_____

_____

_____

_____

_____

_____

_____

_____

_____

_____

_____

_____

_____

_____

_____

_____

_____

_____

Wake Up, Lord. Save Me!

The disciples went and woke him, saying, "Lord, save us! We're going to drown!" He replied, "You of little faith, why are you so afraid?" Then he got up and rebuked the winds and the waves, and it was completely calm."
Matthew 8:25-27

"How long?" I asked. "How long was she under?"

"Five minutes?" the teenager cried. "Maybe more, I don't know!"

I laid my patient on a dry portion of cement beside the pool. The pretty little pig-tailed girl with chubby cheeks and dimples looked to be about eight years old, and as cute as a button, but her lightly freckled face looked dull and colorless, her eyes as lifeless as a plastic baby doll's.

"Is she going to be all right?" her sister exclaimed. "I only took my eye off of her for a minute!"

166

Answering the Call

"Quick," I said tearing open the plastic wrapper for an Ambu-bag. "Get the monitor."

My partner grabbed the EKG monitor and removed the electrode cables.

"Somebody start compressions."

I placed the resuscitator unit over the patient's mouth and gave the bag a squeeze. Her chest rose and fell. Water trickled from the corner of her mouth. One of the firefighters removed his helmet and knelt by my side. He placed his hands on her chest and started pushing against her breastbone with a verbal cadence of one, and two, and three...

"Folks," I heard my partner say, "please stand back. Give us room." He pulled the backing off of a sticky electrode pad and attached it to one of her legs. He repeated the process on each of her other limbs while the firefighter and I performed CPR. "Okay," he said turning on the unit. The EKG monitor beeped. A harsh, erratic, jumpy yellow line traced across the screen. "Let's take a look." He placed a hand on the firefighter's arm. "Hold compressions."

The firefighter stopped. I held my breath. The EKG line flattened out, hiccupped once, and then grew into a regular pattern of uniform complexes. *Oh, thank you, Jesus!*

Why did you ever doubt me? I heard the Lord say. *If I calm the mighty oceans, I can certainly take care of you.*

Answering the Call

I felt elated. I gave our patient two more full ventilations, and then I watched in amazement as she began to cough and choke. We rolled her onto her side, careful to protect her head and neck as the clear pool water drained from her mouth and nose. "Here's oxygen," someone said placing a hissing oxygen mask over the little girl's face. I watched and waited, speaking quietly to her and praying silently as I coaxed her back to life. "Come on," I said. "You can do it. Come on back to us, come back."

She opened her eyes. Her skin turned pink. Then, as if waking from a nightmare and realizing it was all just a terrible dream, she closed her innocent blue eyes again and began to cry. I closed mine too, but I began to pray.

"Thank you," I murmured. "Oh, Lord, thank you so much."

Have you been there? Where the cares of this world make you feel like you're about to drown? Well next time you find yourself in the midst of a raging tempest, with the wind shrieking and waves crashing all around, remember you're not alone. Jesus is right there with you ready to calm the raging storms in your life.

PRAYER

"Lord, I'm struggling. I feel like I'm drowning down here. I can see the surface but I just can't seem to get there. Help me! Give me your hand, Lord. Please save me!"

Answering the Call

APPLICATION

Are you troubled? Are there any problems you can't quite seem to manage? Make a list of some of the storms you have been battling recently.

Read Philippians 4:6-7. In this passage the Apostle Paul encourages you not to worry about these problems. What does he suggest you do instead?

Is there a promise attached to these words of encouragement?

Now read 1 Peter 5:7. What does Peter have to say about anxiety?

Are there steps you can take toward a more peaceful life? A life free of fear and anxiety? Describe how you might accomplish this.

BUILDING BLOCKS OF FAITH

We serve a mighty King. Nothing is too difficult for God.

JOURNAL

_____

_____

_____

_____

_____

_____

_____

_____

_____

_____

_____

_____

_____

_____

_____

_____

I Am Not Ashamed!

"For I am not ashamed of the gospel of Christ: for it is the power of God unto salvation to every one that believeth; to the Jew first, and also to the Greek."
Romans 1:16 (KJV)

"Excuse me," I said looking up at the man. He was huge. Powerful. Broad chest and shoulders clothed in a white karate ghi. And he looked every bit the part, a professional fighter with a knack for breaking bones. In fact he had just broken a pile of concrete blocks…with his head. "Um, Mr. Barlow?"

"Yes?" Frank Barlow turned and looked down at me. "I'm in a hurry, son. How can I help you?"

"I, uh, I just wanted to ask you…" I hesitated and then just blurted it out. "Do you know Jesus?"

Mr. Barlow appeared stunned, caught off guard, but then he chuckled and retaliated as a humored smile broke the stiffness on his face. "Son," he said, "I don't have time for religion right now. I have more important things on my mind."

I grinned sheepishly. I knew I was licked. Besides I didn't know what to say or do next. For that matter, I had no idea why I'd even asked him the question. It was just something I felt compelled to do.

"Okay," I said. "I really enjoyed your presentation."

Mr. Barlow nodded, smiled at me, and walked away. I never saw him again.

A few months later my mother told me a story. She had been at a gathering of Christian women that day, a lady's luncheon of sorts. "We had a guest speaker," she said. "He was a karate expert."

"Really?" I was enamored with the notion of karate. Of black belts and fists. Of breaking boards and blocks and people's heads with nothing but hands and feet. "Who was it?"

"Frank Barlow."

"What?"

"He gave his testimony," she explained. "About how he'd become a Christian. About how he was on his way back to his car after a karate exhibition when this high school kid came up to him and asked him if he knew Jesus."

"Mama, that was me!"

"I know," my mom said with a smile. "I just thought you might want to know you had an impact on his life. He accepted Christ."

Answering the Call

The gospel of Christ is powerful. Life changing. And it's meant for people of all nations—Jews and Gentiles. Everyone.

That was thirty-five years ago. For more than twenty of those years Mr. Barlow operated a dojo in my hometown, called "Judo and Karate for Christ." Today he is a Karate Master, with a 6th Dan black belt in Shorin Jiu Te Do Karate and expertise in numerous other disciplines. But today something else is different about him too…today Frank Barlow knows Jesus.

Are you a Christian? Is there someone you know who needs to know the truth? Then tell them about Jesus. If a skinny eighteen year-old kid can turn a powerful karate expert around by asking him a simple question, then imagine what you could do.

PRAYER

"Lord, if you could use me then, you can use me now. Help me to be as bold today as I was that day. There are plenty of other people out there who still need to know Jesus."

APPLICATION

If you are a First Responder you have frequent opportunities to serve others—to exhibit true concern, to show compassion, and just as important to share your faith in Christ. You see people when they are hurting, seldom at their best. Have you ever felt compelled to share your faith with another person and then failed to do so? Describe a situation where that happened.

Could you feel your pulse increase? Did your hands become clammy and cold? Perhaps you were concerned about how that person might respond, or that someone else might hear you sharing your faith. Describe your emotions at that moment.

Read Mark 8:38. How does Christ say he will respond if you are ashamed of him?

Now read Luke 22:34. What did Christ predict that Simon Peter would do three times before the rooster crowed?

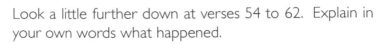

Answering the Call

Look a little further down at verses 54 to 62. Explain in your own words what happened.

Is someone on your mind right now? Write down their name.

Will you commit to pray for this person and then to boldly ask them if they know Jesus Christ?

BUILDING BLOCKS OF FAITH

The Lord is my light and my salvation—
whom shall I fear?

Answering the Call

JOURNAL

What Do You Know?

In the beginning God created the heavens
and the earth...
Genesis 1:1

"You know, you should look at the Milky Way sometime, Bill. Some night when the sky is pitch black. As your eyes begin to adjust and that soft, almost indistinguishable blanket of stars and interstellar gases begins to form, you'll realize you're looking at something far greater than us. Our galaxy! It's over a hundred and fifty thousand light years across. And it contains over a hundred billion stars. And they say it's just one of a hundred billion similar galaxies that move around the universe together. How can that be? How did it all get here? It didn't just happen. You say you wonder if there's a God; I don't. I know there's a God. There has to be."

My friend, Bill, gazed at me and scratched his chin, his computer mind processing the picture and considering it from every angle. He gave a slight nod and then an almost imperceptible shake of his head.

"You may be right," he said. "I don't know. I just don't know."

Answering the Call

The child had curly red hair, a pale freckled complexion, and blue eyes that might have sparkled one day, but it wasn't meant to be. It was his time. Fourteen months old and **already** his time.

Why? I don't know.

When my partner and I arrived the firefighters were already performing CPR. The little boy lay on the ground with his tiny chest exposed. One firefighter's hands pushed against his sternum, another's worked an Ambu-bag pumping oxygen into his lungs at a steady, controlled rate. The mother stood to one side with her hands to her mouth and a stunned expression on her face.

"Oh, Jesus," I prayed as I climbed down from the ambulance. "Lord, please help me. Help me do this right."

My partner and I rushed over to help. I performed a quick assessment and attached the cardiac monitor to confirm a rhythm. There wasn't one. A flat green line traced across the screen. I felt my heart sink. I knew the child was already dead, but I also knew we had to try.

"Good job, everyone," I said trying to keep my cool. "You're doing great. Keep doing exactly what you're doing."

I could tell by their faces that everyone else felt exactly as I did. Confused and scared. A tiny life was slipping away right before our eyes. We all knew our attempts were likely futile. But we held ourselves together. We did it right. Everything proceeded in an orderly fashion, in perfect textbook style. CPR, intubation, IV, drugs—we did it all right. Our Medical Director would have been proud. But despite our valiant efforts the little boy died, and I went home that night wondering why…

"Why?" I prayed. "God, why would you allow this to happen?"

My answer never came.

I used to think I knew it all. Not anymore. I'm not even half as smart as I once thought. All I can honestly tell you with certainty is this: There is a God and He's not me, Jesus Christ died for my sins and I'm going to heaven, and my family loves me. And that includes my dog. Other than that, I just don't know. But the good news is God does know. He made the earth and the moon, the sun and the stars. He even made the fabulous Milky Way Galaxy. He created everything there is. That's what I know, and that's all that matters to me.

PRAYER

Heavenly Father, you created The Milky Way. You created me. You created everything. And that's all I'll ever need to know to trust You with all of my heart.

APPLICATION

Have you ever stopped to consider the immensity of the universe, or the microscopic worlds teeming within a drop of water? Creation occurred. Nothing is here by mere chance. I once heard someone say, "I don't have enough faith to believe this all just happened." I agree with that statement. Read Genesis 1:1…what does the first verse of the Bible say?

Read the verse again. When did it happen?

Turn in your Bible to Job 36:26. What does this verse say about God?

Go to Job 37:5. What does this passage say about man's understanding of things?

183

Answering the Call

Please take a few moments now to read Job 38:1 to 42:3. How does this passage make you feel about God's omnipotence? His understanding?

God created all that there is. He created time. He created you. How should this knowledge affect the way you think about God? The way you respond to His voice?

BUILDING BLOCKS OF FAITH

If God created the heavens and the earth, He knows all there is to know about you.

Answering the Call

JOURNAL

_____

_____

_____

_____

_____

_____

_____

_____

_____

_____

_____

_____

_____

_____

_____

_____

_____

_____

_____

Welcome Home

Therefore, my brothers, be all the more eager to
make your calling and election sure. For if you do
these things, you will never fall, and you will receive
a rich welcome into the eternal kingdom of our
Lord and Savior Jesus Christ.
2 Peter 1:10-11

It was powerful!

Bagpipes played as the horse drawn caisson rolled past an
army of gray-clad Troopers. Upon its carriage deck lay a
flag covered casket that held the body of an old friend of
mine. A true warrior. A brother in Christ—Trooper 352:
Andrew James Stocks, N.C. Highway Patrol.

We called him A. J.

The Caisson moved quietly to the clicking hooves of six
magnificent black creatures, well groomed horses in regal
parade dress, one without rider to signify loss. The horses
stopped. Six Troopers stepped forward and removed the
casket. They marched quietly into the building and set it
in a place of prominence in the front of the church.

Answering the Call

The service was awe inspiring, a beautiful memorial to the life of a true first responder—A.J.: U.S. Marine-Crash Firefighter, N.C. Paramedic, N.C. Paramedic Instructor, U.S. Army Ordinance Soldier, and lastly, N.C. State Trooper. Yes, A.J. dedicated his entire career to the service of others. He risked his life so that others might live and, in the end, gave his life selflessly in the line of duty. He was and still is a true hero.

I felt myself jump at the offering of the twenty-one gun salute. Tears filled my eyes as I heard the bagpipes play and the peaceful closing hymns. But I felt my life change at the offering of the radio report that ended the service. A strong male voice came over the air. I felt confused. It surprised me.

"Raleigh, Troop C—"

Silence fell over the room. At first I thought it was a mistake, someone's radio, a Trooper's handheld crackling to life. But then it came again, crisp and clear, a strong voice from somewhere overhead.

"Troop C—"

Dead silence this time. It wasn't a radio; it was a real dispatch going over the air for N.C. Troopers everywhere to hear.

"Troop C…Attention! Trooper 3-5-2 is 10-42."

10-42…*Ending tour of duty.*

Answering the Call

A. J.'s work on earth was complete, and with that God moved him to his new home in heaven. I know he's there because I asked him one day, "How can you be sure?" He answered, "Because, Pat, I know Jesus Christ died for my sins."

So A. J. has a new home now, and oh what a mansion! Can you imagine it? Built by God's own hands? And it must be marvelous too, for Jesus said, "In my Father's house are many rooms. I am going there to prepare a place for you. I will come back and take you to be with me."

And He did. Jesus came and took my friend home. So wait there for me, brother. Someday Jesus will come to get me too.

PRAYER

"Thank you for my dear friend, A.J. Now give him a rich welcome, Father, into the eternal kingdom of our Lord and Savior Jesus Christ. May his time in Heaven be as meaningful and passionate as his life was here on earth."

APPLICATION

A.J. understood that Christ died for his sins. He repented and received the gift of eternal life, and in doing so secured for himself a room in God's Heavenly home. You have the same opportunity. Read Acts 2:38-39… what does the scripture say you must do to be saved?

To whom was the promise offered?

In Luke 23:32-43 we see a profound example of Christ's free gift being offered to a guilty man. According to this passage, what must one do in order to follow Christ home, to enter the Kingdom of Heaven?

Now read John 14:2-3. According to this passage, where is Jesus now?

Read Acts 1:9-11. What encouragement did the two angels give Christ's disciples regarding His miraculous departure into Heaven?

Answering the Call

God created Heaven; it's His; He owns it all. And no one can go to the Father except through His Son, Jesus Christ. Jesus will come back for his children. Will you being going home with him? Will you receive a rich welcome into God's eternal kingdom, or will you spend eternity wondering where you went wrong?

BUILDING BLOCKS OF FAITH

He who testifies to these things says, "Yes, I am coming soon." Amen. Come, Lord Jesus—Revelation 22:20

JOURNAL

_____

_____

_____

_____

_____

_____

_____

_____

_____

_____

_____

_____

_____

_____

_____

_____

_____

Before It's Too Late!

Therefore, get rid of all moral filth and the evil that is so prevalent and humbly accept the word planted in you, which can save you.
James 1:21

"Medic-7, hemorrhage! A 38 year-old female with a severe laceration. Caller reports *heavy bleeding!* Respond Code-3."

My partner and I didn't need to hear the dispatch twice. We jumped into our truck and drove out of the bay. I pushed some buttons and the ambulance lit up like a Christmas tree, lights flashing, siren wailing—Code-3. Bloody images consumed my thoughts as we raced to the call, and as we walked onto the scene those images came to life—a raucous crowd filled a room decorated with bloody wallpaper and jagged pieces of clear broken glass. My patient stood in the center of the room with a blood soaked towel wrapped around her wrist. Crimson drops fell from her fingertips and splattered onto the floor.

I reached for her arm to remove the towel.

"No," someone shouted. "Don't take it off!"

193

Answering the Call

"Relax," I said. "I need to see the wound." But as I removed the last of the towel I realized I had made a mistake. A bright red stream spurted from the severed artery, shot across the room, and sprayed the far wall with crimson-colored paint. "Quick," I shouted to my partner. "Hand me a dressing!"

Like my patient, our nation is hemorrhaging. Losing the core values that once made us great. As a people we have become saturated with moral filth. Where are we headed? Will we survive or will God turn His back and leave us to fend for ourselves?

My partner handed me a trauma dressing and a bandage roll, and within seconds I had the wrist tightly wrapped. But the bleeding was far from controlled. Blood continued to drip from her fingertips. Her skin continued to pale.

"Let's go," I said to my partner. "This bleeding must be stopped…before it's too late!"

A moment later we had her in the back of our ambulance with the lights flashing and the siren wailing again—Code-3. I tied the tail of the bandage to the overhead railing hoping that elevating her arm would lessen the flow of blood, but it didn't. I tried using a pressure point, pressing my fingers against the artery above the wound, but the blood still flowed. I had one more option. I wrapped a tourniquet around her arm and tightened it. Finally the bleeding stopped.

Answering the Call

Is there any dirt in your life? A dark secret or hidden sin? If so your spiritual life is hemorrhaging, keeping you from a closer walk with the Lord.

After starting a large bore IV and administering a fluid bolus, I called the ER to notify them of our arrival. The doctors were waiting for us when we arrived, gloved and gowned in surgical scrubs, ready for business.

"Be careful," I said as an eager resident stepped forward. "This thing will shoot across the room if you take the bandages off."

"Relax," he said with a chuckle. "I got it."

I shrugged and watched him remove the tourniquet. The blood soaked dressings began to drip. He began removing the bandage. I left the room. I couldn't watch.

I returned a few moments later to find an empty room. But the gurney, the floors, the walls—they were covered with blood.

It's time you applied some direct pressure. Get rid of the moral filth in your life. Confess your sins to God. Because once hemorrhage starts it's mighty hard to stop. Humble yourself and turn your face to God…before it's too late.

PRAYER

"Heavenly Father, I have sinned against You. Plug my wounds. Stop my spiritual hemorrhage. Help me to live a life that is pleasing and honorable to you."

APPLICATION

How do you think we're doing? As a people? As a nation? Can you list several problems common in our society that are indicative of spiritual hemorrhage?

How about your life? Are you spiritually healthy? What areas of your life could use some hemorrhage control?

What do you believe is to come of our nation if we fail to turn from the path we are now following? What will become of you?

Read 2 Chronicles 7:14. What three things does God say we must do if He is to forgive our sins and heal our land?

What steps will you now take to live a life more pleasing and honorable to God?

BUILDING BLOCKS OF FAITH

Uncontrolled hemorrhage kills the body. Uncontrolled sin destroys the soul. Learn to master sin, otherwise it will master you.

JOURNAL

_____

_____

_____

_____

_____

_____

_____

_____

_____

_____

_____

_____

_____

_____

_____

More Inspirational Books From
❧ **Christian Devotions Books** ❧
www.christiandevotionsbooks.com

Answering the Call -
Inspirational Devotionals from a Tested Paramedic
by Pat Patterson   **Price: $9.95**

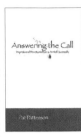

Jesus said, "Greater love has no one than this, that he lay down his life for his friends." The First Responders in your community do just that. They sacrifice comfort and safety to protect the lives of others, always waiting, and always wondering when they will find themselves answering the next call. This book was written for them, but it applies to anyone who searches for courage and hope, struggles with a difficult relationship, or suffers through pain or loss. Are you seeking a closer walk with God? Wondering what comes next? Answering the Call can help you find your way. It reveals the simple truth that Jesus Christ is Lord, and that to follow him is to find true meaning in life. Christ... the First Responder, is calling you now.

Will you be answering the call? "The promise is for you and your children and for all who are far off -for all whom the Lord our God will call." - Acts 2:39.

Learn more about this book at: www.answeringthecall.us

Faith & FINANCES:
In God We Trust, A Journey to Financial Dependence
by Christian Devotions contributors   **Price: $9.95**

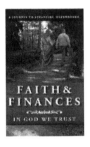

Jesus spoke about money and material possessions more than he talked about heaven, hell, or prayer. He noted the relationship between a man's heart and his wallet, warning, "Where your treasure is, there your heart will be." This contemporary retelling of the Rich Young Ruler brings a fresh look at the relationship between a person's faith and their finances. Within the pages of Faith & FINANCES: In God We Trust you'll find spiritual insight and practical advice from Christy award-winning writer Ann Tatlock, plus best-selling authors, Loree Lough, Yvonne Lehman, Virginia Smith, Irene Brand, DiAnn Mills, Miralee Ferrell, Shelby Rawson and many more.

Great faith calls us to trust God, not our wealth. Read how others have cast off the golden handcuffs and learned to live the abundant life Jesus promised in this contemporary retelling of the Rich Young Ruler. Faith & FINANCES: In God We Trust, A Journey to Financial Dependence - turning the hearts of a nation back toward God one paycheck at a time.

Learn more about this book at: www.faithandfinances.us

Spirit & HEART: A Devotional Journey
by Christian Devotions contributors   *Price: $9.95*

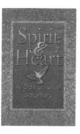

What is a devotional journey? It is the Bible. Today we enjoy the benefit of the prayers, wisdom, praise and sorrow of people who, during their lifetime, chose to remember the times God worked in their lives. That is devotion to God and dedication to recording "His Story." The daily devotions included in this book are heartfelt stories, lessons, and advice from others who have traveled the devotional journey. This book is a primer, a tool to get you started on the path toward spending your best moments with the Father. Christ says, where your heart is there your treasure will be. Treasure His words and whispers as you walk in the footsteps of award-winning authors Ann Tatlock, Loree Lough, Yvonne Lehman, Virginia Smith, Irene Brand, Shelby Rawson, Eddie Jones, Cindy Sproles, Ariel Allison-plus many more.

Learn more about this book at: www.devotionsbook.com

Emerson The Magnificent!
by Dwight Ritter   *Price: $12.99*

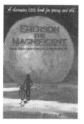

"A charming little book for young and old."

How an old bike takes a young man for the ride of his life.

"What a delight... though I thought it unlikely that a bicycle could do much to unravel some complicated issues, my skepticism was outvoted. It really doesn't matter how old you are, Emerson talks to you. Dwight Ritter's illustrations made me smile as much as his story warmed my heart. Emerson's message challenged my thinking, then threw me a lifeline, reeled me in and rescued me. Get it! Read it! Give it to everyone you know! " - by Pat Lindquist.

Learn more about this book at: www.emersonthemagnificent.com

**More Inspirational Books Available From
Christian Devotions Ministry's Book Division
www.christiandevotionsbooks.com**

Love Hina

the novel

Story by
Kurou Hazuki

Art by
Ken Akamatsu

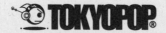

HAMBURG // LONDON // LOS ANGELES // TOKYO

Love Hina: the novel
Written by Kurou Hazuki
Illustrated by Ken Akamatsu

Translation - Anastasia Moreno
English Adaptation - Craig Spector
Copy Editor - Eric Althoff
Design and Layout - Jose Macasocol, Jr.
Cover Design - Christian Lownds
Editor - Kara Stambach

Supervising Editor - Nicole Monastirsky
Digital Imaging Manager - Chris Buford
Production Manager - Jennifer Miller
Managing Editor - Lindsey Johnston
VP of Production - Ron Klamert
Publisher and E.I.C. - Mike Kiley
President and C.O.O. - John Parker
Chief Creative Officer and C.E.O. - Stuart Levy

A 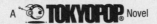 Novel

TOKYOPOP Inc.
5900 Wilshire Blvd. Suite 2000
Los Angeles, CA 90036

E-mail: info@TOKYOPOP.com
Come visit us online at www.TOKYOPOP.com

ISBN: 1-59816-445-7

First TOKYOPOP printing: April 2006
10 9 8 7 6 5 4 3 2 1
Printed in the USA

CONTENTS

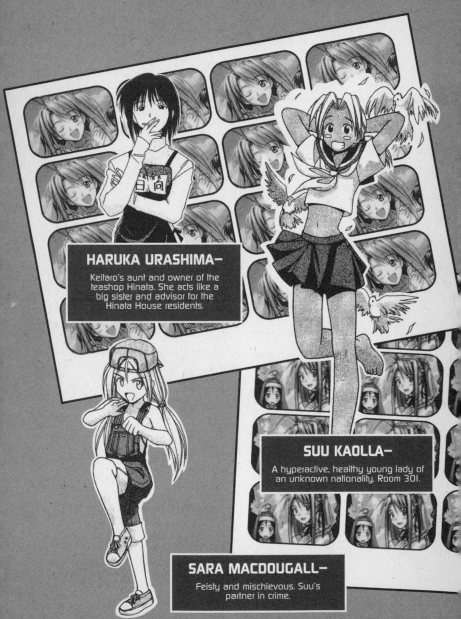

Love Hina

HARUKA URASHIMA—
Keitaro's aunt and owner of the teashop Hinata. She acts like a big sister and advisor for the Hinata House residents.

SUU KAOLLA—
A hyperactive, healthy young lady of an unknown nationality. Room 301.

SARA MACDOUGALL—
Feisty and mischievous. Suu's partner in crime.

CHARACTER INFORMATION

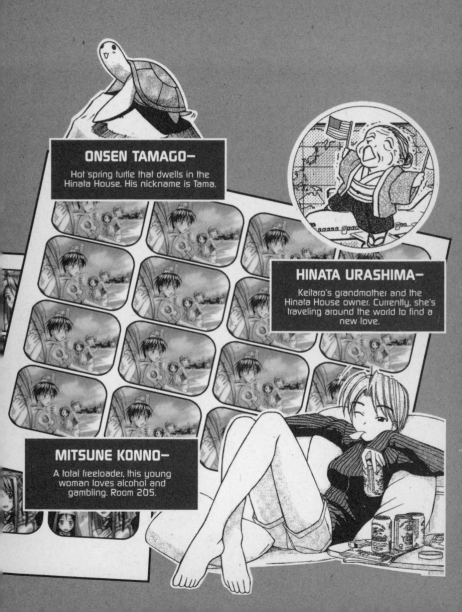

ONSEN TAMAGO—
Hot spring turtle that dwells in the Hinata House. His nickname is Tama.

HINATA URASHIMA—
Keitaro's grandmother and the Hinata House owner. Currently, she's traveling around the world to find a new love.

MITSUNE KONNO—
A total freeloader, this young woman loves alcohol and gambling. Room 205.

Love Hina

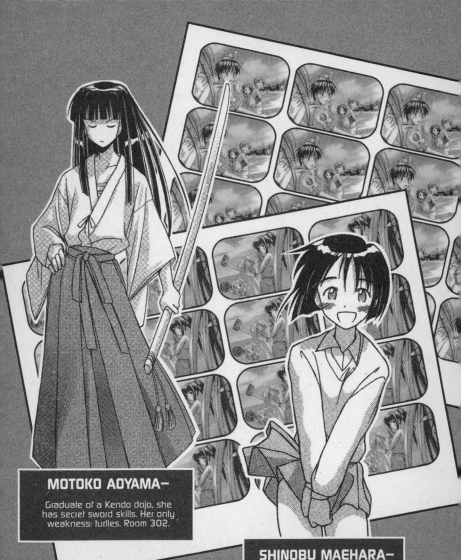

MOTOKO AOYAMA—

Graduate of a Kendo dojo, she has secret sword skills. Her only weakness: turtles. Room 302.

SHINOBU MAEHARA—

A shy, innocent, domestic engineer. Room 201.

CHARACTER INFORMATION

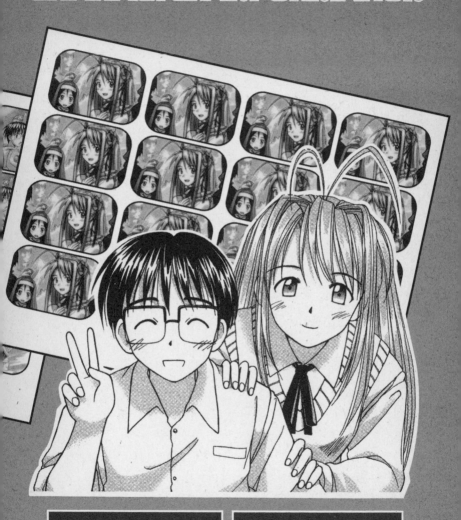

KEITARO URASHIMA–

Hinata House manager. Sole male among the females. He's studying to enter Tokyo University.

NARU NARUSEGAWA–

A bright, energetic, pretty young lady, also aiming to enter Tokyo University. Room 304.

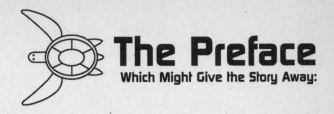

The Preface
Which Might Give the Story Away:

Thank you for waiting patiently, *Love Hina* fans! We are finally able to present to you the novelized version of *Love Hina!*

I am the scriptwriter for the anime, but this novel is based strictly on the original manga, so please understand that none of the new, original characters that were created solely for the anime will be used in this story.

I tried to stay as true to the original setup of the manga as possible, but nevertheless, I'm sure hardcore fans of *Love Hina* will find many inconsistencies. But, please understand, writing this was really tough!

Even as I plotted out the novel, the manga series continued on. I had to diligently avoid similar plot points

and changed settings, particularly regarding making the Hinata House a hot springs inn, and the secret of the inner lawn's old annex, etc. etc. When things got sticky, I called Akamatsu-sensei to resolve any overlapping issues and timeline inconsistencies.

"Akamatsu-sensei, in the first volume, Haruka refers to Keitaro as her nephew, but isn't she Grandma Hinata's granddaughter? Shouldn't they be cousins?"

And then Akamatsu-sensei would laugh and say, "Well, I'm not sure why she called him her nephew. Ha ha ha!"

We were going around in circles!

With so many unsolved riddles in *Love Hina,* some of the story elements shifted around, and things got lost in the gray zone. There's a good chance that certain parts of the novel will differ from the later manga volumes.

The premise I'm operating on now is that all of the characters and settings adhere strictly to the original story.

And so, without further ado, it's show time!

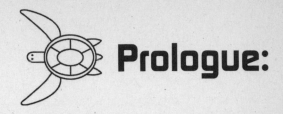 **Prologue:**

Okay, I have a confession: I don't get girls.

No, wait—I don't mean I don't *get* girls, even though that's technically true, it's not like I've ever *had* one or anything—I mean I don't understand them. I don't understand the way they think or feel. I have no clue what they think about me, except maybe that I'm a giant pervert.

Okay, now you're looking at me funny. Let me explain.

Ever since I was a little kid, I never really talked to girls much. The only woman in my life at that time was my mom. She was the head of the family and she also ran our old, traditional Japanese candy store.

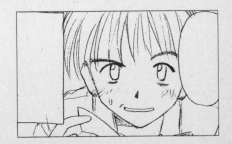

I don't mean to disrespect her, but she ran that shop like a Marine drill sergeant. (And come to think of it, she kind of *looked* like one, too.) So, it was extremely difficult to wrap my young mind around the concept of femininity, based solely on her example.

Of course, all the schools I went to were coed, so there were plenty of girls in my classes. But I was way too scared to talk to any of them. And if any of them ever bothered to talk to me, it was to say things like, "Keitaro, go sit over there!" and they'd point to the farthest seat in the cafeteria. Or they'd say, "Keitaro, give us your homework!" usually followed quickly with, "Keitaro, the answers are all *wrong!*"

Then they'd punch me in the nose.

Well, no, wait . . . that wasn't the *only* thing girls ever said and did to me. I mean, if that was the sum total of my experience with females, that would be just too pathetic, right? So, there had to be something nice that a girl said to me, at least once. Right?

Gimme a second . . .

I'm thinking . . .

Er . . . Um . . .

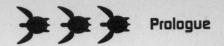

Hey, no pressure, okay?

Nope, I got zip. My only memory of the female sex involves tears, bruises, and the scent of floor wax (due to landing face-first one too many times).

Story of my life, folks.

Hang on—something's coming to me. It's real faint, like a flashlight flickering on and off in my mind. There's a girl . . . she's crying . . . and there's a scarf . . .

Ah, yes. It was in third grade, right after winter break. The back of the classroom had these little shelf spaces, aligned in alphabetical order, for each student to put gym clothes, books, and craft tools in. My shelf space was usually empty, but that day I noticed a gift. It was wrapped in *Liddo* paper. Liddo was a popular television anime character back in the day. I really liked the tenacity of his personality, but my friends always made me pretend to be the professor, because I had glasses.

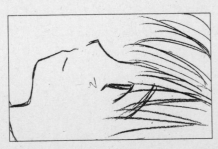

I digress.

Back to the wrapping paper. Inside was a typical hand-woven scarf. It was kind of nubby, like something your granny would give you. But it came with a little card, on which the words *I made this just for you!* were scribbled in girly, loopy script. There was even a little heart at the bottom.

At first, I thought someone left the present behind by accident. I looked around the classroom, but no one seemed to pay any attention. Then some of the boys noticed, and they said, "Oooooh, Keitaro got a scaaaaaaarf!"

And then I wondered: did this mean I was popular with girls?

Could I possibly have—*gasp*—a secret admirer?

I was totally psyched! I kept the scarf wrapped around my neck the whole day. Of course, the heaters were running full-blast, and so in retrospect, that probably wasn't the smartest move . . . I was going for "dashing," but pretty soon I was sweating like day-old cheese. But I just figured it was a small price to pay for being studly.

I kept it on no matter what the teacher said, or how much I dripped. When I went to the restroom, I tied it on extra tight, so it wouldn't fall off. I almost choked to death,

but it didn't matter. I was a stud muffin. I was the man. Someone seriously dug me.

But who?

By the end of the fourth period, I could feel someone's eyes boring into the back of my head. It was a little girl. She never really talked to me (just like all the other little girls) but now she was glancing at me a whole bunch. I reasoned that the scarf had to have come from her.

So, you were the one who gave me this present, I thought. *I'll treasure it, and even though I never noticed how cute you were until just now, I'll care for you, starting today . . .*

I looked deeply into her eyes, and it was like I could almost hear her say, *Thank you, and please take good care of my heart!*

After school, I stayed behind, looking for that little girl. Suddenly, I heard someone cry behind me, "You thief!"

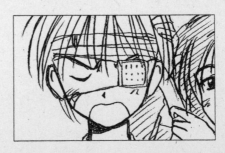

Then, *crunch!*

A fist whacked me, right in the nose!

I turned around, and saw the little girl had tears glistening in her eyes. For a moment, I thought she was worried about me, but she frowned. She hid behind the boy that had decked me—Urasawa, whose shelf was right next to mine.

Urasawa glared at me. "How do you think she feels?" he barked.

Oh. The riddle was solved. This little girl had put the gift in my box by mistake. Now Urasawa was sticking up for her. It was clear from the way she clung to his coat that she really liked him.

Of course, she could have just said the scarf wasn't for me, or told me to give it back. Why did she just look at me silently all day? How could I have possibly known what had happened? Was I supposed to be psychic?

Kids, myself included, could be so cruel at times. What Urasawa said sounded so grown-up and totally righteous that I instantly got labeled as the school villain. Other kids in class spread rumors, and from that day on, I was the boy who "didn't get girls."

Sometimes even the *teachers* would nonchalantly comment in classes, "Keitaro, now I heard you don't get girls. You can't become popular like that, you know."

Like they'd know popularity if it bit them on the behind!

After that, I just took it for granted that I didn't get girls.

But that didn't stop me from trying! I even took the entrance exams for Todai (Tokyo University) three times (to major in literature) all because of a promise I'd made to a girl before I ever entered kindergarten.

See, once I'd met a beautiful little girl. We played together in the sandbox.

"Did you know?" she asked suddenly. "If two people who love each other very much go to Tokyo University . . ."

"Love?" I interrupted, confused. I gulped.

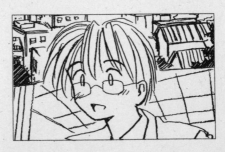

"They'll live happily ever after!"

I paused, mulling that over. Happily ever after sounded good. "Hm."

She smiled at me. "When we grow up, let's go to Tokyo University together!"

Before I could say anything, she kissed me!

My mind went blank at that very moment, and it stayed that way. I don't remember anything about that kiss, except the slight sound of lips smooching my cheek. (That was a sound I wouldn't hear for the next twenty years of my life, you see.)

The idea of Tokyo University was planted in my brain that day, and it took root. Once I figured out that Todai meant Tokyo University and not *to-dai*, a lighthouse, getting into Tokyo University became my life's goal. It wasn't because I'm completely lame and think that all childhood promises should be kept. It's because I'm too lame to think of anything else to aim for.

I never saw that little girl again. I can't remember her name, or what her face looked like. She's probably forgotten all about that promise. But I remember.

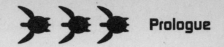

I'm still a guy who doesn't get girls. And I'm still stuck here, at the very place where I'd made that little girl our promise—at the Hinata House.

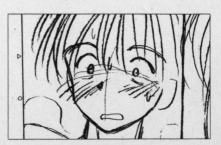

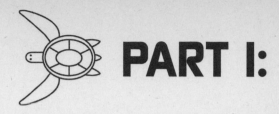

PART I:

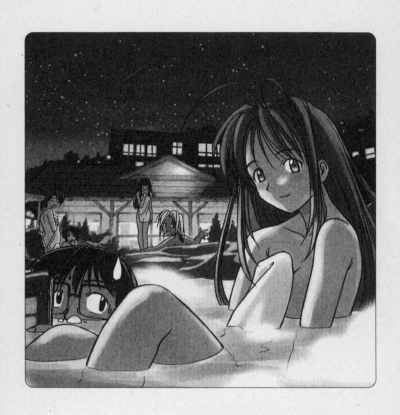

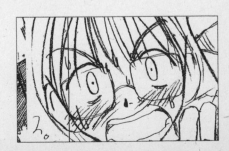

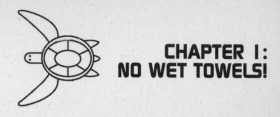

CHAPTER 1:
NO WET TOWELS!

I had a dream. The kind of dream you might hesitate to tell others about.

Tama, the Hinata House's pet turtle (some might say resident) clung to me. He clung, and then he slithered . . . all over my body.

"Whoa, whoa, stop!" I cried. "That tickles, Tama!"

But he ignored me and continued on his journey, releasing some sort of squishy substance as he moved. The tickling sensations turned into something more . . . um . . . serious. As Tama slipped past my armpit and slid down my side, I thought, *No, don't go, stay there and do the squishy-squishy like that* . . . Oh well. It was weird, but it felt kinda good, and this was just a dream, okay?

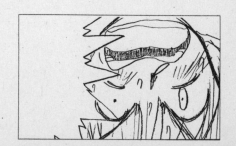

Tama kept moving, slithering across my chest, my stomach, and down toward . . . well . . . *there*. I was lost!

Please don't go down there! If this continued, I'd get labeled as the only guy in the world who ever got off on a hot springs turtle. I pictured my name, Keitaro Urashima, in the *Guinness Book of World Records* under "Weirdest Crazed Sex Fiend."

Now, all I had to do was move away from Tama, but I couldn't make myself budge. Tama kept crawling lower, and I started getting a little hot. I convinced myself that it was only because Tama's squishy substance was heating up. When Tama's nose was just about to touch me—wait, this is getting gross, right?

Hey, I thought of a stupid pun: "The hot springs turtle was about to touch my hot turtle!" I pictured that as the front-page headline of tomorrow's paper.

"Tama, no!" I pleaded, yanking the waistband of my pajamas back. But it wasn't Tama down there after all—it was Naru!

Naru Narusegawa was an eighteen-year-old girl, two grades younger than me. She was way cute, with long brown hair (a few strands of her bangs stuck out like

little antennae; she was so adorable!) and big brown eyes, plus she had a majorly hot body. Also, she was extremely smart. She ranked number one in Japan for the National College Entrance Preparatory Exam—but for some odd reason, she failed the actual entrance exam on her first try.

My feelings for Naru were . . . well, secondary, really, because, at the moment, instead of Tama slithering around in my pants, there was a pint-sized Naru down there!

She smiled up at me and said, "Myu!"

I woke instantly, and then cursed myself for missing out on what could have been a damn good dream. I was so shocked by the teensy Naru in my pants, that I hadn't really taken a good look at her, but now I remembered, she was naked!

Maybe I can see her again if I go back to sleep, I reasoned. But then, I felt a distinctly odd sensation. There really *was* something crawling all over my body!

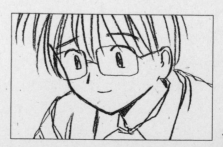

Whatever it was, it felt both painful and ticklish at the same time.

"Am I still dreaming?" I mumbled.

But no—I looked up at the ceiling panels and saw some light leak through the cracks. I lived in Room 204, the manager's room, and Naru's room was right above mine. There was a giant hole in the ceiling, always had been, and when she moved in, Naru patched it up with wooden boards, but sometimes, late at night, I could see her lamps' light filter through the cracks. Those times, it felt like we were the only people in the whole world, and that made me happy.

So, the fact that I could see the ceiling in such detail and remember all that about Naru, I figured I had to be awake. But what the hell was crawling around my back and calves?

Finally, I peered down and noticed a bulge in my futon. Well, naturally—that dream was kind of exciting. Unfortunately, this bulge was too big for *that*. While I was thinking about bulges, the crawling sensation turned into scratching. It felt like someone was plucking the fine hairs off my legs!

"Ouch!" I yelled. I tucked up my legs and winced.

Then, I heard girls' voices: "Oh no, he's awake!"

"Almost there! We need to go up!"

I recognized those voices! I watched with something akin to horror as the bulges in my futon grew. "What are you doing?!"

I ripped back the covers and saw two girls, each one holding magnifying glasses, infrared scopes, duct tape (with some of my freshly plucked hairs attached), a laptop computer, and various other gadgets. They clung to my legs.

"Suu? Sara?" I called. "What are you doing in here?"

Suu Kaolla and Sara MacDougall were Hinata House residents. Of course, they didn't room together. Sara lived by herself on the second floor of the Hinata teashop, in fact. At the moment, it was well past midnight, so I couldn't fathom what they were doing here.

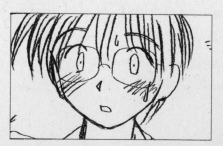

"Suu, you're not sleepwalking, are you?" I asked.

Suu was a light sleepwalker, and without (her roommate) Motoko Aoyama's supervision, she could sometimes wander into other people's rooms and fall asleep there.

The mischievous duo seemed reluctant to spill the beans, but finally Sara said, "We were actually . . ."

"Actually, what?" I pressed.

"We came to *yobai.*"

I stared blankly at them. I was trying to make sense of Suu's Japanese (she had a very thick accent). Possible kanji combinations of the word yobai could mean good multiple, four times, drunk-crawl (were they crawling around because they were drunk?) . . . And then the final meaning for yobai—to have sex—flashed through my mind like a giant, blinking, neon sign.

"What?" I screeched.

"No! We were really trying to—mmphmmt!"

Sara quickly covered Suu's mouth and hissed, "Don't tell him, stupid! Just say we're here to yobai."

When Sara eventually pulled her hand away, Suu immediately asked, "Does a yobai taste good?"

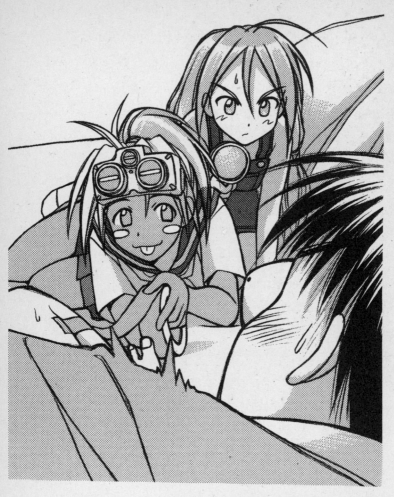
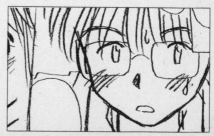

Sara grimaced. "Forget it. Just use that thing while I distract him!"

"Roger!" Suu agreed.

They whispered to each other. I couldn't make it out. I was too busy thinking about yobai. Suu was still in junior high, and Sara was in elementary school. There had to be a misunderstanding. They probably didn't even know what yobai really meant, the silly girls. I mean, Suu always said she really liked me, and even though Sara punched and kicked me all the time, that was just her way of letting me know she cared. Whatever they were doing to my legs probably caused me to have that erotic dream, but, honestly, I couldn't really have feelings for girls their age (although, admittedly, Suu's arms, legs, and breasts were developing nicely).

But I knew better than to even go there or think that! I mean, sure, it was entirely possible that I'd never be approached this way by another girl in my entire life . . . and Sara was from the open-minded United States . . . and Suu was from somewhere south . . . maybe these girls were more sexually aggressive than Japanese girls? I mean, if they both pounced on

me and I accidentally responded to their seduction, it wouldn't be my fault, right?

Suddenly, arms wrapped around me. Sara clung to me!

I could feel the blood drain from my face. I twitched and mumbled to myself, "Stay strong. Stay strong."

"Hey, he's saying something," she said to Suu. "His eyes are glazing over."

"Sara, the secret weapon is all set up!"

"Oh! Ready, set, go!"

Suu pulled out an odd machine with a *doki* (a large ceramic piece) that twirled around. (She was always inventing cockamamie machines.) She released it, but the ceramic piece kept twirling. It headed straight for me, going *GWOM-GWOM-GWOM*.

Was yobai supposed to involve machines? If that contraption machine hit me, I had a feeling it would hurt.

"Hey, this thing's safe, right?" Sara asked, worried.

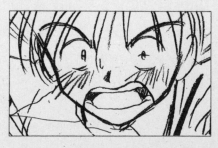

"He'll just pass out," Suu replied.

I won't just lose consciousness, I thought, *I'd die!*
"Eeeek!" I shrieked.

CRUNCH!

Naru lifted up the wooden boards, jumped down the hole, and crushed the machine with a flying kick. The whirling doki machine sprawled along the tatami mat, little pieces bouncing over her feet.

"Oh, no! My invention," Suu said wistfully.

"Forget about the invention!" Naru said, frowning. "Sara? Suu? What are you two doing here so late at night?"

The girls solemnly bowed their heads. That was a tad strange, because they usually didn't calm down when Naru scolded them.

"Oh, thank God, Naru!" I said, relieved. I stood up and brushed some debris off my shoulders. "I was about to get killed!"

Naru just glared at me. I looked down and realized why—my pajama pants were halfway down!

She raked me with her gaze. "So *that's* what's going on."

"Wait, you're getting it all wrong," I blurted out. (This is what always happens.) "Look, I was just about to get killed—"

"So you dragged two girls into your room," she interrupted, "pulled your pants down, and turned on some strange machine! I see how it is!"

"Na-Na-Narusegawa . . ." I stuttered.

"I've had enough of you!" And then, *WHAM!* Naru lashed out with her Naru Punch—a killer right hook that broke the speed of sound and sent me soaring through the sky. "Pervert!"

The next thing I knew, I flew so high up into the air that the Hinata House looked like a distant star.

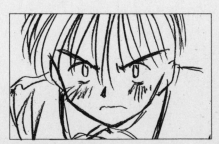

The Hinata House had a hallway that connected the south side to the north, where the baths were. It was the end of August (much too hot to concentrate on our studies) so we had agreed to take a swim in the outdoor pool to try and cool down.

I tried to explain to Naru once again what had happened last night. This time, she actually listened, and when I was done, she just said, "What a strange story."

She took off her glasses (she only ever wore them to study) and smiled. She looked fabulous no matter what she wore, but when she took her glasses off, I thought she was stunning. I considered all the Hinata House girls my friends, but Naru was special. She was the cutest, and we got along well (when she wasn't punching me) but that wasn't the only reason she was special to me.

Anyway, it was really important to me that Naru didn't get the wrong idea about me. I didn't want to be cast as the villain all over again. And Naru, well, she was always really quick to judge me, instantly assuming the worst. "Keitaro is up to no good again," she'd say, and then dish me up a Naru Punch or a Naru Kick or, my personal favorite, a Naru Backhand.

I honestly believe that Naru was just trying to keep the peace. But she didn't really trust me. The last time we went to the beach, we seemed to have such a good time together. But last night, she looked at me like I was some sort of disgusting maniac. I just don't get girls.

I did my best to tell her my side of the story, but she still had some questions.

"If Sara and Suu wanted to mess with you, they would have come in and barreled straight at you, right?"

Barreled was right. But Suu's Flying Knee Kick and Sara's infamous ambushes had me sporting bruises and scratches year-round.

"And if the girls were really messing with you," she continued, "they would have just come out and said so. I think they might be hiding something."

Naru stared at me. I couldn't help but think of the dream last night, when the pint-sized Naru sucked on my body with her soft tongue, and slithered . . .

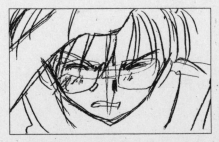

"Oh, not here, Naru, everyone can see . . ." I murmured, lost in dreamland.

"What?" she asked. "Are you even listening to me?"

I shook my head, banishing that particular fantasy, and nodded furiously. "But, other than messing with me, why else would they come to my room?" I scratched my head. "Maybe they really *did* want to sleep with me."

Naru folded her arms and raised one eyebrow. "You think you're such a stud, huh?"

I blushed. "Sorry."

"Did they do something to you?"

"I don't know." I shrugged. "They were using infrared scopes, so maybe they were looking for something. They plucked my leg hairs, so, I dunno, maybe they were trying to make a clone? I wouldn't put it past Suu, that's for sure."

Naru laughed. "Why would they want to clone a perverted freak like you?"

I bristled. "What are you so worried about anyway? It's not like you care," I said.

Suu and Sara always played tricks on me. This was the first time it ever turned me on, though. It was just weird to have Naru so obsessed with the subject.

Her expression hardened. I wondered if I'd said something wrong. She started walking, and I followed, trying to think of something to say.

"Just how far are you gonna go?" she asked, spinning around.

"Huh?" We'd reached the entrance to the Hinata House's main bath. It was for women only. (But as manager, I have to clean it, mind you.)

"Ah ha ha, I thought we'd do a few laps together, you know."

Naru ignored my joke and disappeared into the changing room.

I worried I had made her mad, but, hey, it wouldn't have been the first time.

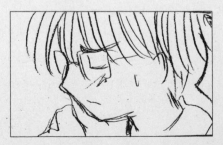

A set of stairs led up to the men's bath. Actually, it wasn't a men's bath, but a small, old drying room (used to air out futon mattresses from the north tower) that had a little wooden tub, barely big enough for one person.

From here, you could almost make out the main bath, which had big, beautiful rocks and waterfalls and reflecting pools, but most of the view was blocked by large trees. Once, when I was trying to get a peek, I leaned too far off the edge of the balcony and fell. Why am I telling you that?

The reason the men's bath is banished so far away from the main bath is simply because I'm the only man around. I moved here over a year ago, when my parents stopped financially supporting me (I'd just failed the Todai entrance exam for the third time). I was flat broke, so I rolled into Grandma's Inn. I'd had fond childhood memories of the place, and I couldn't think of anywhere else to go.

But when I dropped by, Grandma Hinata wasn't in. She was on vacation, traveling the world in search of new love. The old Hinata Inn transformed into the Hinata

House, which became an all-girls dormitory.

My aunt, Haruka, ran the Hinata teashop, and she'd told me then about the plight of the Hinata House. The place was in desperate need of a manager. It so happens, I was in desperate need of a place to live. So out of great sympathy for the girls' plight, I agreed to become the resident manager.

Hey, it's a paying job and a place to stay, and I'm surrounded by beautiful young ladies. The only bad thing is, and I'm not making excuses, but . . . the girls here loved to party, and that really cut into my study time. Oh, it's not like I was ever *invited* to the parties or anything, but being surrounded by a bunch of loud, happy, gorgeous girls is kinda distracting.

Once again, I failed to get into Todai. I didn't just fail; I *flunked*. Somehow, Naru managed to flunk too. So we both had to study for an extra year. A whole year. Sometimes I wondered if the little girl who I'd made the promise to even

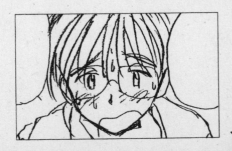

existed, or if she was a figment of my imagination. But, it didn't matter so much anymore. Getting the chance to go to Todai *with Naru* was fast becoming my secret desire.

Of course, if I ever said that to Naru, she'd say she wasn't studying just to go to college with me, and then she'd probably punch me.

I couldn't tell if she liked me or hated me, half the time. And why was she so stuck on whatever Suu and Sara were up to? "Gosh, I really don't get girls," I blurted out.

"Want me to teach you, pal?" said a sultry voice.

I jumped up. I *knew* that voice.

It was Mitsune Konno, but everyone called her Kitsune (fox) because she was so foxy. She placed her hands on the tub and peered over the edge at me. "Oh, you're so naughty, you'll get me all wet!"

She was only a year older than Naru. They'd known each other since elementary school. They were polar opposites. Naru was a perfectionist, a very serious honor student, and a modest girl. Kitsune loved men, dirty jokes, alcohol and gambling. Plus, she was a total free loader.

Once I had remarked on how she and Naru were totally different, and Kitsune had commented that they

were both similar in that they had killer bodies.

It was true; they were hot. But Naru was nice, and Kitsune was nasty (the kind that keeps you awake and leaves you frustrated).

Naru's moods were easier to gauge—she yelled or cried openly. I never could figure out Kitsune. I had no idea what she was doing here, and it made me nervous.

"Kitsune . . . th-th-this is the *men's* bath," I stammered.

"I know that," she whispered. "I thought I'd scrub your back for you."

She raked me with her gaze. She'd probably rake me with her *tongue,* if I wasn't careful. I stood up—then covered my privates and ducked back down into the bath.

We stared eye to eye. Kitsune batted her eyelashes.

"What's up, Kitsune?"

"Nothing. I just can't hold back anymore." She

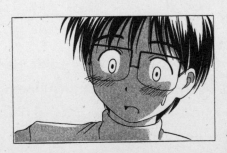

stood up and stripped off her tee shirt. Her breasts almost bounced out of her bra. "My clothes are all wet. But if I take off my bottoms, I'll be naked."

"W-w-wait! Please don't do that!" I panicked.

She smiled. "Will you let me scrub your back?"

"Um. Okay?"

As soon as I saw Kitsune strip down to her underwear, the lower half of my body got excited. I felt flushed and dizzy.

"I can stay in the tub, right?" I asked. I wasn't about to get out just to get scrubbed down.

"My, my, already?" she murmured. "Oh well." She chuckled at my predicament, then grabbed a washcloth and started to scrub my shoulders.

"Um, Kitsune?"

She didn't reply. I could feel her hot breath on the back of my neck. It shivered down my spine and gave me goose bumps. Originally, my arousal had been kept in check because I was nervous, but now . . . I shuddered.

Kitsune was very pleased with herself. And had to be excited as well, she was breathing so heavily. Was it

possible that a girl could get aroused just from the sight of my naked back? Her breath felt like a long fingernail stroking up my spine; it drove me wild!

"Can you stand up?" Kitsune's voice sounded so . . . normal.

"It's already up."

"What a lame joke," she said. "Just stand up!" She grabbed me under my armpits and hauled me to my feet.

"Oh, it's embarrassing!" I covered myself, but Kitsune just squatted down, her face almost brushing against my butt. I mean, I'm talking just a few millimeters of space between us, here!

I turned my head, and saw she wasn't aroused in the slightest bit.

"Kitsune, what are you looking at?"

She startled and hastily looked up. "What do you mean?"

"You're looking at me so hard. Do I have a mole or

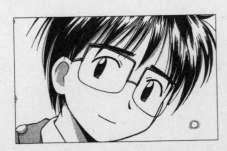

something there?"

She gasped. "I don't see any, but . . . I can tell your fortune by reading moles!"

I just stood there, very confused. "Uh huh."

"Let me read your future for you, Keitaro," she said. "Turn around, show me your front."

"Wait! Front, as in . . . *front?*" I gulped. I started babbling.

She just whipped me around. "Don't worry. Just let me look."

"But I'm naked," I whined.

"I can't see your moles with your clothes on, silly! I already said, I can't hold back anymore!"

Just then, I heard the voice of a goddess. (My goddess, at least.)

"Kitsune, is that you?" Naru called.

"Yeah!" Kitsune called back.

I felt faint. Naru walked into the men's bath and my goddess transformed into a demon from hell. "What the hell . . . ? Keitaro, you dirty little weasel!"

"No! No, Narusegawa, I—"

Kitsune tried to make a hasty exit, but Naru stood in

the entrance (wearing nothing but a towel, I might add).

"What are you doing here?" Naru asked Kitsune. "Did Keitaro drag you in here?"

Kitsune hid behind the tub, using me as a human shield. I wobbled a bit.

Naru covered her eyes and screeched. "You freak! Don't show me that dirty thing!"

I frowned. *"Dirty?* I'm in the bathtub, for crying out loud!"

"Don't get near me, you pervert!" Naru's face turned bright red. She grabbed the lip of the tub and pushed it over.

KER-SPLASH!

The tub flipped. Water poured down onto the lawn below, taking me along with it.

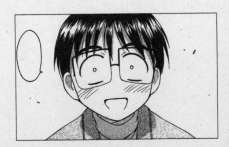

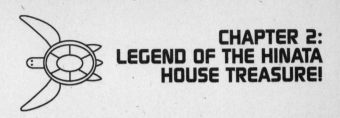

CHAPTER 2:
LEGEND OF THE HINATA
HOUSE TREASURE!

"**A**h-ah-ah-CHOO!"

Shinobu watched me sneeze, a worried expression on her sweet face. "Are you okay?" she asked.

Not really. I had been left out on the lawn for some time. Even though summer wasn't over, my body was thrown out of whack from being naked, wet, and exposed to the open air.

Now I lay in my room, helpless, certain I was coming down with a cold.

The only girl who spoke to me on a regular basis was Shinobu Maehara. She attended the junior high school nearby. She was somewhat shy and a

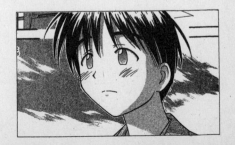

little nervous, but man, when it came to household matters like laundry and cooking, she was a real pro. She made the Hinata House feel like a home. Shinobu was definitely the type you'd want to bring home to meet Mother.

At first, she was a little wary of me, but now she was kind to me. She smiled easily now. I came to think of her like a baby sister.

"Shinobu, did you hear anything?"

"About what?" She couldn't look me directly in the eyes; she seemed so flustered.

"Do you know what Kitsune and the others are up to?"

She shook her head emphatically. "I don't know anything about the secret treasure hidden somewhere in the Hinata House!" she blurted out, then clasped her hand over her mouth.

"Treasure?" I repeated.

She bit her lip and looked extremely regretful. "Kitsune and the girls said it." She leaned forward and whispered, "There is a hidden treasure on these grounds!"

"That's impossible," I told her gently. "If there was anything buried here, this old inn would have been torn down years ago to get to it."

Honestly, I had no clue what all the fuss was about. Grandma Hinata was vacationing around the world, so she had to have *some* sort of fortune, I supposed. But these old buildings and the idea of "treasure" just didn't mix.

"Anyway, what does treasure have to do with me?" I asked.

"I don't know," Shinobu said, shrugging. "They didn't tell me anything other than not to tell you."

This was mighty puzzling. "I wonder if they thought I'd take it away from them or something? Are they trying to seduce me so I'll let them keep it?"

Shinobu looked at me like I was a specimen under a microscope. "Did Kitsune do something odd to you, Keitaro?"

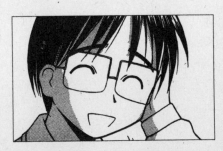

"Yeah! She stared at my naked butt, for one!"

Shinobu flushed. She wrung out the damp towel in her hands. Water droplets splashed on the tatami floor. "You showed her your . . . your . . ."

"I didn't *show* it to her. She looked at it all by herself!"

"No way! That's just so filthy!" Shinobu screwed up her face until she looked like a little pink raisin. "I didn't know you and Kitsune had the kind of relationship where you'd show each other your . . ."

"We *don't*," I scolded. "Don't get any funny ideas, Shinobu." I reached out to pat her on her knee, but she inched back. She leaned so far back that I could see her panties (pink, with teddy bears on them).

"Keitaro?" Shinobu looked at me, worried again.

I felt something warm drip down my upper lip. I had a nosebleed!

"You're not doing so well, Keitaro."

"No, I'm all right," I insisted. "Perfectly fine!" *Oh, man, I'm going to hell for thinking bad, bad thoughts.*

"Oh dear," Shinobu said. "I must have said something troubling to you! It's all very shocking."

Shocking? What was she talking about? "Why?"

She blushed beet-red and flailed her arms a bit, looking adorably flustered. "You and Kitsune, I mean. . . Naru probably didn't like that, so she flipped the tub . . ."

I shook my head. "Naw, Naru just got pissed that I exposed myself to her, is all."

She frowned. "I don't think that's the case."

Man, I really don't get girls. I had no clue what Shinobu was talking about. Why would Naru care if I showed my body to Kitsune?

Something caught my eye. I crawled slowly toward Shinobu to get a better look.

"No, Keitaro!" She backed away. "What if someone walked in? Your body . . ." She froze, looking horrified.

I hugged Shinobu and said, "Please scoot over."

She lunged to the side, and I stepped forward to examine a black spot on the wall. At first I thought it was a bug, but it was too shiny. It was a tiny camera lens!

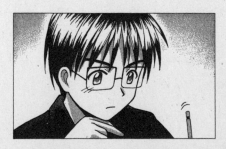

Shinobu and I spent the next half-hour debugging my room. There were over a dozen CCD cameras—each one had Suu's trademark on it, so there was no doubt in my mind who was the culprit.

But why would she want to spy on me? This was the sort of thing perverts put in the stalls of women's restrooms, or the paparazzi use to get pictures of famous stars. I knew that Kitsune, whose room was next to mine, had poked a hole in the wall to check me out while I studied with Naru, so I figured she was up to something. But I had no idea if she dragged Suu and Sara in on the spying scheme.

Then again, maybe I'd turned into a stud, and hidden videos of me had become a must-see Internet item . . . *Keitaro Uncovered! Keitaro After Dark! Keitaro Gets a Naru Punch!*

Um, okay, maybe not. Maybe I should just *ask* what was going on.

I left the room in search of Kitsune, but only got about three feet before I stopped short. A long, sharp blade gleamed under the hallway lights.

"Urashima. Quit sniveling and accept my challenge to a duel!"

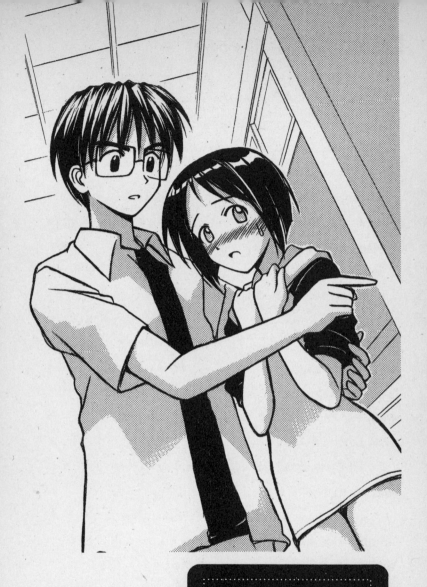

成瀬川なる編
NARU NARUSEGAWA

I recognized this blade—it was the sacred sword of the Hinata House, *Shisui*. Motoko Aoyama wielded it. She was a one-of-a-kind character, extremely unique even among the girls at the Hinata House. She carried a katana replica, and wore ceremonial Japanese clothing (actually, she wore the *hakama,* the traditional samurai outfit) all the time, except when she went to school. And she *hated* men. Or at least, she hated *me.* I was the only man at the Hinata House, and so I did the math.

She would resolve even the most minor incident with her sword, no questions asked, and no quarter given. Rumor had it that Motoko had studied the *shin mei ryu,* the secret sword fighting style. She could do serious damage, no doubt about it.

From what I could see, Motoko was as tall and slender as a supermodel. She had long, jet-black hair (a rarity these days) and a pretty, angelic face. If she'd allow it, guys would fall all over themselves for a girl like her. But she insisted that she was studying the ways of sword, and therefore she refused all worldly pleasures, including love relationships. *Especially* love relationships.

Last time we went to the beach, Motoko stopped being so formal, and opened up to me a little. But now . . . well, I was one of those wimpy males she despised the most, anyway.

When Motoko pointed a real katana (not a replica, like she used for practice) at me, wimpy male that I was, I obliged her request to go to the large drying room upstairs. (Unlike the small drying room that doubled as the men's bath, this was a bigger room at the other end of the hall.)

Motoko stood next to some sheets and towels that were hung up to dry; they wavered gently in the breeze. I stood next to the doorway, so that I could run for my life, should the need arise.

"Urashima."

I shivered. "Did I piss you off? Let me tell you, the thing with Suu and Sara was *not* my fault! They attacked *me!* And Kitsune? I had no idea what she was up to . . ."

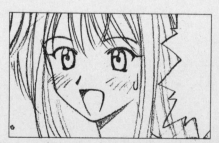

Yeah. I was babbling. You try keeping your cool when Motoko points a katana at you.

"Urashima!" she yelled loudly.

I shut up.

"I have no wish to waste lives," she said harshly. "So take your clothes off," she mumbled.

". . . Huh?"

She swore under her breath. "Just do as I say and take off your clothes. All of them!"

I frowned. "What's wrong, Motoko? I'm not hiding anything . . ."

"Don't make me say it again, Urashima."

I whimpered. "But I'm catching a cold . . ."

"Take them off!" She waved her sword around. She was so wound up I worried she might explode.

What's a man to do?

"Okay, okay! Sheesh. Everything, right?" I unbuttoned my shirt.

Motoko stared at me the whole time, which was mortifying. I unzipped my pants and dropped them unceremoniously to the floor. Finally, she looked away.

"Hurry up. What's taking you so long?" she hissed.

"I'm done," I said.

Technically, I wasn't completely naked. I didn't take my underwear off, and my feet were freezing so I kept my socks on, but I was ready to die of embarrassment.

Motoko rolled her eyes. "How dare you show that to me!"

I frantically ran behind the sheets, shouting, "But you insisted I take my clothes off!"

"Zanma ken!"

I gulped. *Zanma ken* was a technique used to dispel demons, wasn't it? "Is my body some sort of monstrosity?"

SWASH!

Motoko swung her sword, slicing the sheets to shreds. I freaked out.

"Calm down, Motoko, calm down!" I slipped behind more sheets, but Motoko drew nearer with

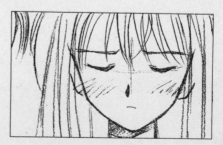

each swing, reducing all the linens in her path to white confetti.

I was cornered. The only place I had yet to go was the roof, but Motoko would kill me before I could ever reach it.

"Get a hold of yourself! Are you seriously trying to kill me?!" I bellowed.

Motoko had a blank, hollow expression. It didn't matter what I said, she wasn't listening to a word of it. She had demanded I remove my clothing, but she couldn't stand the sight of me, and just lost it.

I had to find a way to snap her out of it, but words were no good, so . . . I distracted her by throwing my underwear at her.

"Ura . . . shi . . . ma . . . What . . . ?" Motoko froze. As if she were a puppet on a string, her left hand jerked up and removed my underwear from her face. She inspected them, and then turned purple and screamed, "URASHIMA!!!"

I'd never seen anyone so furious.

She rushed toward me, her sword swinging down— suddenly a shadow passed between us. Someone stood in front of me.

"Narusegawa?" I squeaked.

For a second, I thought Naru had come to save me, but she immediately turned around and cried, "Die, you perverted scum!"

She whacked me a good one. Once again, I flew into the sky.

Later, Naru actually took pity on me. We sat in Shinobu's room, eating some *manju* (sweet bean cakes) that Shinobu had prepared. Without a doubt, Shinobu was the best cook in the house, and I was starving, what with all the energy I'd used up the last few days just trying to survive.

As we munched, Naru grilled me mercilessly.

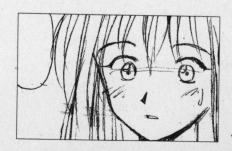

"And then what did Motoko say?"

I shrugged. "She refuses to come out of her room. I heard her reciting some sutras."

"Well, that makes sense, since she saw that thing." Naru sighed.

"What do you mean 'that thing?' "

"You know. *That thing* is *that thing*. I sure didn't expect to have to see that thing twice in one day." She shuddered.

Oh. *That* thing. "You jumped into those situations all by yourself! For all I know, you were *trying* to see my thing!"

She wrinkled her delicate nose. "Knock it off! Why would I want to see your filthy naked body anyway?"

"Then . . ." I scratched my head. "Then, why did you come? First you walked in on me with Suu and Sara, and then later with Kitsune and Motoko. Why?"

Naru paused. She exchanged glances with Shinobu, then turned back to me and glared. "Because those girls were all in danger!"

I folded my arms and sighed.

"If I let a horny animal like you all alone with those girls, naked like that, who knows what kind of trouble they'd be in!" she said.

I wasn't about to argue that, technically speaking, *I* was the one in danger, with my butt hanging in the breeze each time. I figured Naru was trying to preserve the peace and protect the other girls. She didn't care if anyone saw my naked body. I guess I sorta hoped she'd be a little jealous and possessive of me, but that was just a silly fantasy.

Shinobu looked like she wanted to say something, but she just shook her head and asked, "Why do you think everyone's acting so strange lately?"

That's the reason the three of us had gathered in Shinobu's room—to figure out what had gotten into Suu, Sara, Kitsune, and Motoko. Even as we wondered, Suu and Sara lurked just outside Shinobu's window, waiting to pounce on me. It was starting to get really creepy.

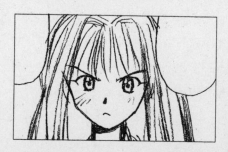

"First I thought Suu and Sara were just messing with me, but if Kitsune and Motoko are involved, it goes deeper. The objective always seems to be—"

"Your naked body," Naru finished, disgusted.

"You don't have to say it like that," I told her. "I have no clue what they want with me."

"I can't imagine," Naru muttered.

"So, you're saying you wouldn't want to look at my naked body, Narusegawa?"

"No way!"

I was frustrated, but there didn't seem to be any recourse, so I reached for another one of Shinobu's manju. Unfortunately, Naru had the same idea, and she snatched it up first and took a big bite.

"Aw, that was mine," I complained.

"Hush," Naru said. "You hear that?"

We all went quiet, listening intently. Voices were whispering just outside.

"I've had enough," I said loudly, like a bad actor. "I'm going to take a walk outside!"

"Why are you raising your voice like that?" Naru asked, frowning.

I winked at her. "Let's go for a walk, you guys." I pulled both girls out into the hallway and acted like we were walking away, then quickly hid behind the door. Shinobu and Naru caught on, and stayed quiet.

Less than ten seconds later, the window opened. Suu and Sara snuck in. Sara carefully looked around, but Suu, in typical Suu-fashion, went straight for the manju.

"There's almost none left!"

"Forget that," Sara said. "We have to follow them!"

"No need," I said, emerging from my hiding place.

Sara pulled Suu up short. "Oh no! We gotta go!"

"But . . . manju!" Suu pouted.

"Suu," I said pleasantly. "I'll give you some manju, but first, you have to tell me what you're up to."

Suu's eyes lit up at my promise, but she hesitated. "Kitsune warned us not to tell you . . ."

"I'll give you as much manju as you want!"

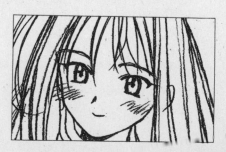

"Deal!" Suu, predictably, switched sides without hesitation.

"Oh. I didn't think that would work," Shinobu whispered. "Well done, Keitaro!"

Naru huffed. "It's not hard for him to think on her level."

We traded seven manju cakes in all, to learn that the Hinata teahouse was at the root of this whole mess. So the three of us decided to get to the bottom of everything by speaking to the teashop owner—my aunt Haruka.

"Well, supposedly we had an incoming phone call." Haruka held a cigarette between her fingers as she casually explained.

Aunt Haruka was pretty cool, and usually nice to me. Sometimes she acted like a referee between the girls and me.

"Yesterday, I left the store for a while and had Kitsune cover the phone, and that's when Grandma called."

"Grandma Hinata?" I asked.

"Yeah," she said. "Anyway, Grandma mistook Kitsune's voice for mine and told her something. Kitsune got all excited and starting yelling words like 'treasure' and 'riches' and 'important thing' . . . She had kind of a crazy look in her eyes."

"Treasure?" Naru and Shinobu repeated simultaneously.

I was astounded. Grandma Hinata started this crazy treasure rumor? That was just so weird.

"What's all this about?" I asked, folding my arms. What did Grandma say to Kitsune, exactly?

Haruka just looked at me like I'd grown two heads.

"Do you know what she was talking about?" I pressed her.

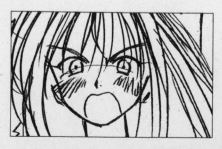

"How the heck should I know?" She shrugged. "If there really was treasure, she'd have told me by now."

Knowing Aunt Haruka, I'm sure Grandma would have been hesitant to share assets with her, since Haruka had a tendency to make dangerous investments. But I chose to sip the coffee she'd given us, instead of voice my thoughts.

I gulped. The coffee tasted really strange.

"Is something wrong, Keitaro?" Shinobu asked.

"Kaaaaah!" I said, coughing. I felt like I was breathing fire. Sweat gushed off me in torrents. My stomach started convulsing wildly, burbling ominously.

I jumped up and ran to the bathroom. I barely made it to the toilet in time. I ripped off my clothes, but still felt feverish. My tummy made weird *boogly boogly* noises.

In the midst of my agony, I had the funny feeling someone was watching me . . .

"Tsk, tsk. Gotcha!"

I looked up. Kitsune was braced up on the ceiling like a ninja. She jumped down nimbly and kicked my clothes into the corner.

"Did you make that coffee, Kitsune?" I asked, pained.

"No, but I tossed in tons of hot peppers and laxatives, along with Suu's medicine," she said simply. "I figured if I made you hot and sick, you'd take off your clothes whether you wanted to or not!"

I grimaced, covering myself. "Are you trying to kill me?!"

She waved her hand. "Oh, you'll be all right."

"What makes you think that?" I asked through gritted teeth.

Kitsune ignored me, lifting up my legs to get a look at the soles of my feet.

"What the hell are you looking for?" I demanded.

"Well, you know," she said absently, inspecting me closely. "It's like I said, I love you so much, I can't hold back anymore."

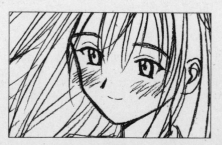

It was such an obvious lie, but I was stupid enough to wish it were true. I guess most guys would feel the same.

"I want to know every inch of your body," Kitsune purred. "So, Keitaro, do you have any tattoos?"

I rolled my eyes. "No!"

"Hm." She cocked her head to the side. "I've heard about a white powder tattoo that only shows when you're in a hot bath. But I don't think that's it."

"What are you babbling about?" I asked tiredly.

Kitsune's arms wrapped around my knees like two slithering snakes. She forced my legs open and pressed her face close to my thing. I flushed, embarrassed.

"That's so funny. Where is it?" she mumbled. "Oh, hey, maybe you need to get hotter. What makes you hot? What if I do this?"

She straddled me, grabbing the back of my neck and pushing my face into her cleavage. Her soft bosom and heady perfume were, I have to say, heavenly.

"How's that? Are you getting hotter? Maybe it'll show up now."

"What the hell?" I said, but my voice was muffled and it came out more like, "Whuddahellmmph!"

Kitsune wriggled. "Quit talking! It's really ticklish—and I'll get hot too!"

She bounced up and down playfully, but for me, it was just excruciating. I yanked my face away, gasping for air, and said, "I have no idea what's going on!"

"Like that makes a difference!" she said, grabbing my head and pushing it farther into her cleavage. I was going to choke to death (and I have to admit that it would have been a happy way to go) but I wasn't ready to die just yet.

Kitsune continued to purr and coo. "Say, Keitaro, you know about your grandmother's call, don't you?"

"Mphmagamcalmmph?" It was really hard to hear, my head half-buried in her bosom like that.

"Your grandmother said she forgot a really important treasure that she'd hidden long ago. She asked me to find it, so I asked her where it was."

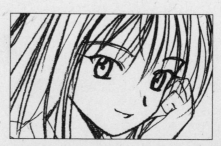

Kitsune moved my head around, rubbing against me. It was torture, I tell you.

"She said it was 'Keitaro's secret' but then Haruka came back, and I was so startled that I accidentally hung up the phone!"

Suddenly, someone knocked loudly on the door. I heard Naru say, "Hey, Kitsune, are you in there?"

"Hold on, I'm almost finished," Kitsune cheerfully called back.

She continued to move my head around as she said, "Your grandmother's treasure was a secret, and she hid it somewhere inside the Hinata House. But she forgot to take it with her on her trip. And since the treasure is your secret, I figure its whereabouts have to be written on your body somewhere!"

I finally managed to escape her clutches and raised my head to gulp in some air.

She pouted. "You didn't have to stop!"

I huffed. "What do you mean, my secret?" I had no recollection of anyone writing anything on my body, ever. Granted, my memory wasn't the best, but that's not exactly something I'd be likely to forget.

Kitsune bounced up and down on my lap, her breasts jiggling right in front of my face. "Let's find the treasure together! If it belonged to Grandma Hinata, then it must be really valuable! How about we split the fortune, and run off to a foreign country!"

I wasn't really interested in treasure. I kinda liked living like a bum at the Hinata House. If I was going to fantasize about running off to an exotic place (like New York, Shanghai, or Rio de Janeiro) I'd only want to go with one other person. I could see it all so clearly—an expensive, lavish apartment. I'd sit on a plush sofa, in my silk smoking jacket, a glass of warm brandy in my hand. Naru would sit down next to me. We'd gaze out of the large windows at the gorgeous landscape. She'd be wearing a glamorous, low-cut dress. I'd slip off her spaghetti shoulder straps, and then lean down and . . .

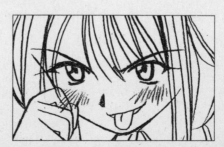

Okay, I had to stop. Fantasizing about sleeping with Naru while Kitsune straddled my lap and Naru banged on the door just outside was a life-threatening situation.

I forced myself to calm down. "Living in a foreign country might be nice."

"I know, right?" Kitsune winked at me. She pulled me close . . .

CRACK!

Naru had punched a hole in the wall, big enough to stick her head in. Her face was red, and she looked ready to kill me.

"What might be nice?!" Naru yelled.

I tried to wriggle out of Kitsune's grasp, but she just held me tighter.

"Don't bother us now, Naru, it's just about to get better!" Kitsune giggled.

There I was, my pants around my ankles, Kitsune sutured to my waist, and Naru about to kill us all.

Suddenly Aunt Haruka came up behind Naru and said, "Whatever. But who's gonna pay for the damage to the wall?"

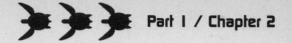

Naru and Kitsune both froze.

Just then, my stomach rumbled loudly, and I cramped up something fierce. "I think you'd all better leave!"

Wisely, the girls fled.

A little while later, we reconvened in the teashop, my embarrassment now—pardon the pun—behind me. We chatted about what to do with Grandma's strange request. Kitsune was convinced there was a map to whatever "really important thing" Grandma had hidden somewhere on my body.

Shinobu offered, "If you want to find the treasure, Keitaro, I'll help." (But help meant that she had to check out my entire body.)

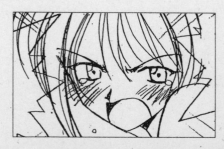

Haruka made the logical suggestion, "What if we just call Grandma again?" She got up and went to place an international call, but there was no answer. She tried several different numbers, but no luck.

"Hey, Keitaro, if you find the treasure, I get dibs too," she said, as if Grandma had passed away and we were divvying up parts of the estate. (Money makes people evil, for sure.) "I read in an historical novel that a tattoo can appear when a person dies."

I wondered if she would really kill me?

Naru glared balefully. I could sympathize— anyone who had to see my naked body that many times in one day would be upset. But since none of it was my fault, I thought she needed to chill out a little. I tried to talk to her, but she was deep in thought and ignored me.

She told Shinobu and Aunt Haruka that she was leaving, and then stood up and made her way back to the Hinata House.

I chased after her. "Narusegawa. Hey, Narusegawa!" I finally caught up to her. "What should we do? Do

you really think there's any treasure? I think Kitsune misunderstood. But if there is a fortune, that would be great! I could be a millionaire! If that happens, let's go somewhere fun!"

Naru turned around. "I guess going to Todai would just be ridiculous, if that were the case."

I sobered. "No, it's not. I was just saying all that stuff 'cause I know it'll never happen."

Naru sighed. "Come on." She grabbed my arm and headed toward the cafeteria.

"Where are we going? Can't we talk in your room?"

"Just come on!"

Naru pushed me all the way to the cafeteria, then locked the door behind us. All our rooms were built in the traditional Japanese style, so we didn't have any locks. Motoko and Naru installed simple locks when they moved in, however, and the cafeteria doors were altered when the inn became a dorm, because

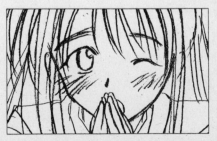

knives and natural gas and other dangerous stuff was kept here.

She turned the lock, and kept her back to me. I didn't know what to do, so I leaned against a chair and waited. But several tense moments passed, so I said, "Narusegawa? Are you okay?"

"Strip," she commanded.

I couldn't believe my ears. "What? You . . . Now?"

"I said strip!"

My overactive imagination once again got the best of me. I pictured Naru saying that to me, then throwing herself into my arms. Except she was wearing a wedding veil, garter belts, and sexy lingerie, as if this was our honeymoon . . .

All my memories of Naru flashed before my eyes at that moment—the time we stayed in the same lodge during the Kyoto trip—when we first met in front of Tokyo University on that snowy Christmas day—the first time we kissed, at the beach (okay, so that was accidental, but it still flashed before my eyes) and then finally—the vision of Naru's beautiful, creamy skin, which I got to glimpse all those countless times I entered the women's bath by mistake . . .

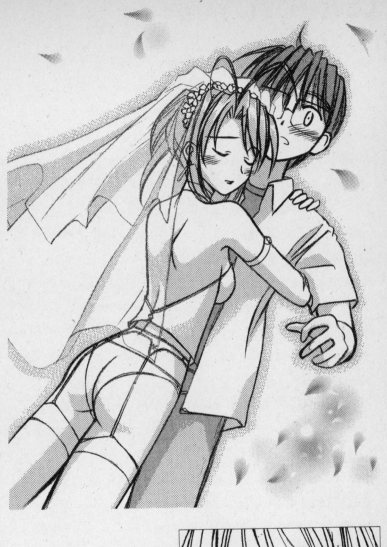
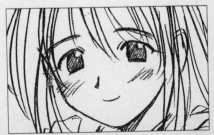

Everything had been heading in this direction . . .

I grabbed my pants, then pretended to hesitate. "But Naru, why are you in such a hurry? There's no ambiance in the cafeteria."

"You don't need any ambiance."

I was shocked. So, she was just after my body? *You don't need my heart, Narusegawa? I don't want that kind of relationship, then.* Yet, I still kept removing my pants.

"Narusegawa," I said, gulping, "this is actually my first time."

"This is my first time too, looking at a guy completely naked."

Naru was sooooo cute! "I'll do my best," I promised.

"You don't need to do a thing."

What? You're going to lead me the whole way through? Huh, could be kinky.

"Are you ready?" Naru turned around. She had put her glasses on. I was a bit disappointed, because she's much hotter when she doesn't wear them.

As she approached, I asked, "Shouldn't you remove your glasses?"

She cocked her head. "But I can't see clearly without them."

Oh, you want to see my face when we . . . You want to look into my eyes and . . . I placed my hands on her shoulders and thought, *No accident this time. This will be a real kiss.*

I closed my eyes and went to hug her gently. But my arms grasped thin air. Naru had squatted down and was looking intently at my thighs.

"Narusegawa?"

"There doesn't seem to be anything unusual there," she said, as if she were inspecting a Petri dish. She frowned. "Never mind."

"But . . . Huh?!"

Naru looked up, and I finally caught on. She was simply looking for the treasure map, like everyone else.

"Uh, you don't have to look for the map, Naru," I said quickly, trying to cover my blunder.

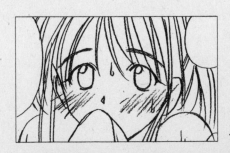

Naru remained emotionless as she examined my legs. I was glad I hadn't removed my underwear yet.

"You want to find the treasure, right?" she asked. "Since you can't find it yourself, I'll do it for you."

I shook my head. "It's okay. We don't even know if it really exists."

Naru frowned. "What do you want to do? Ask Kitsune or Motoko to check for it? Or Suu or Shinobu?"

"I don't know!" I flailed my arms. I didn't like this at all. I had imagined a thousand possible scenarios with Naru kneeling at my feet, and none of them were like this. I couldn't stand the fact that Naru could do this and remain so detached. I picked up my pants from off of the floor and forcefully stuck my right leg in.

Naru tried to stop me. "I haven't finished."

"Yes, you have. Forget it."

"Why? Why can't it be me?" She looked like she was ready to cry.

"I don't want *anyone* to check out my body!"

"Do you hate me looking at you?"

I sighed. "Do you want the treasure that badly?"

Naru's entire expression changed. She just shut down. I had no clue what she was thinking. But if all she wanted was the treasure, then I would be hurt.

"I don't need any stupid treasure," Naru spat out.

I folded my arms. "Oh, is that so? But you were checking me out real good."

"You bastard!" Naru raised her fist.

I yelped and braced for a Naru Punch, but it never came. When I opened my eyes again, I saw that Naru had lowered her fist.

Slowly, I reached for the rest of my clothes and put them back on. Suddenly, the door shook violently. It sounded like grinding metal . . . A sword tip poked through the crack.

SNAP! The lock broke, the door flew open, and Motoko barged in, Shinobu at her heels.

"What's going on?" I asked.

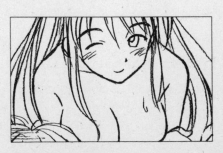

"I sensed you were troubling Naru, and I see now that I was correct!" Motoko replied, blushing an angry red.

"No, no," Shinobu quickly countered. "I just wanted to start cooking dinner, but the doors were locked, so I asked Motoko to open them." She smiled, looking at Naru and I. "Nothing bad happened, right, Keitaro?"

I quickly nodded, but Naru just stepped outside without a word. *Great, now they'll all get the wrong idea,* I thought. Luckily, Shinobu and Motoko let it drop and left to prepare dinner.

I finished dressing, wondering how many times my clothes were going to come off today.

Eventually, Motoko murmured, "I apologize, Urashima."

I'm sure Motoko couldn't stand the uproar over the Hinata House treasure hunt, and she just wanted to find the "important thing" as soon as possible so people would stop talking about it and life could return to normal. Typically, Motoko needed order and discipline in her life.

"Besides," she said, her cheeks still red, "I'm sure it's gross to have people keep checking you out like that."

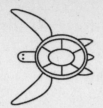

CHAPTER 3:
NARU AND KEITARO, ALONE

That night, I checked my body from head to toe. I didn't believe Kitsune completely, but since we still couldn't reach Grandma Hinata, we had to pursue all possibilities.

I'd never checked out my body so closely before. Weird creases and curly hairs stuck out in my mind. I ended up finding absolutely zip. I checked every crack and crevice, but there was no tattoo, no moles, no odd blotches, nothing on my skin. I decided I'd tell everyone the news at breakfast, and so I just went to sleep.

But the next morning, I startled awake when someone entered my room. I looked up. Haitani and Shirai, my former schoolmates, stood over me.

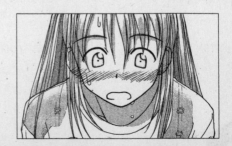

"What the hell are you doing here? And so early?"

"No biggie," Haitani said, peeking closer at my legs.

I quickly tucked them up under my blankets and narrowed my eyes.

"We're your friends, right?" Shirai said, grinning like a cat about to catch a canary. "It's been a while since we hung out with you, Urashima."

"Yes, a while," Haitani agreed, snuggling closer to me.

"We just went to the beach together, remember?" I said.

"Oh, really?" Shirai asked and faked a laugh.

"No way." Haitani looked me up and down.

I sighed. "There's no treasure map!"

They both laughed. "What are you talking about?"

I just stared at them until Shirai broke down and confessed, "Well, yesterday we bumped into Sara downtown. She mentioned there might be a clue on your body."

Man, Shirai and Sara were both blabbermouths.

"We didn't take that story seriously," Haitani rushed to explain.

"Uh huh."

About three seconds later, both of them pounced on me and pinned my arms and legs down. "Help!" I cried. "Someone, help!"

Kitsune poked her face in the room and smiled. It was really unusual for her to be awake this early in the morning. She took one look at my classmates and glared suspiciously.

Haitani and Shirai let go of me immediately and exclaimed, "Hi, Kitsune!"

"What's going on?" she asked.

"Oh, we thought you could help us with something . . ." Shirai started.

". . . So please make us your slaves," Haitani finished.

But Kitsune wasn't exactly impressed. She turned her head and called out, "Suu? Sara? Do it!"

Like ninjas, the two girls jumped silently into the room. Almost faster than the eye could see, they

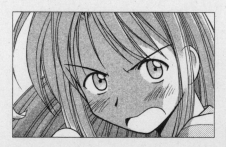

tied beanie hats with little turbo-powered propellers to Haitani's and Shirai's heads. The propellers spun furiously and the two guys floated up to the ceiling, drifted out of the window, and flew away.

We ignored their screams. I was sure they'd be fine.

Kitsune sat down with a serious expression on her face. "If those two heard about it," she said, "then a lot of tourists visiting the hot springs will probably want to come looking for the Hinata House treasure too."

"I'm sorry. It's all my fault," Sara said sorrowfully.

"It's in the past," Kitsune reassured her. "We need to think about how to deal with the here and now."

Seeing how serious these girls were about finding the treasure, I started to feel a bit guilty. Sure, it was fun having them chase after me. Of course, all the man-handling and having to constantly get naked was annoying, but part of me enjoyed the attention. But it was time to end this, once and for all.

"I checked my own body out last night. Didn't find a thing."

Kitsune frowned. "This calls for emergency action."

Everyone except Naru had gathered in the cafeteria. According to Shinobu, when Naru heard about the emergency meeting, she just sat at her desk and continued to study.

I took a deep breath. "Even if lots of people have heard about the treasure, I'm sure most of them don't think it's real. In order to rule out whether Grandma had anything important hidden away or not, please, I need someone to check my body out one last time."

Everyone traded concerned looks. Aunt Haruka raised her hand. "Ah, Keitaro . . . It would be pretty sick

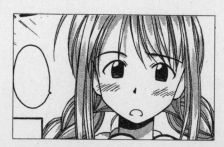

if all of us took your clothes off and checked you out together."

I nodded. "Agreed. You girls should do a drawing. That way only one girl, picked at random, will check me."

They all frowned. "Why?" Suu asked.

Suu and Sara were the only ones who opposed my idea. Suu explained that she had made a new invention that could scan my entire body. But, since it was nuclear-powered and there was a high probability it would explode (like so many of her inventions) we quickly rejected that option.

"Let's stop wasting time. Just knock him unconscious," Sara suggested, lunging at me. But she accidentally tripped over Tama, who flew up and bounced around, landing on Motoko's neck.

"The turtle! The turtle!" Motoko whispered, horrified. "Get it off!"

Motoko hated turtles. She swung her katana around like a crazy person.

Kitsune and Haruka just poured themselves some *sake* and sat back to watch the show. Shinobu ran around, trying to calm Motoko down, while Suu and Sara just giggled.

I rested my chin on my hand and smiled. No stopping the party now.

The drawing took place that afternoon.

Haruka and Motoko had both gone to bed early, and Kitsune was so drunk she couldn't see straight, so the remaining three girls drew straws.

"Oh dear, it's me!" Shinobu said, looking a little queasy.

Suu and Sara laughed at her and dubbed her "Keitaro Urashima's Official Body Checker-Outer."

I sighed. I was a tad worried about such a young, innocent girl staring at my naked body, but what else could be done? I led her to my room with mixed feelings.

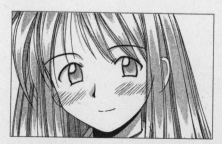

"Can you see anything?" Sara whispered from behind the room's partition.

"Hee hee, Shinobu and Keitaro look like they're going on a pre-arranged date."

I opened the door, but they both hopped on one of Suu's inventions and bolted away. I glanced back at Shinobu, who looked seasick.

"Shinobu, you don't have to do this if you don't want to."

"No, I'll do it," she said, trying to be brave. "Please let me do it."

I nodded and sat down beside her. We stared at each other for almost ten minutes in excruciating silence. Every time I noticed someone behind the partition, I shooed them away.

Shinobu's face alternated between blushing red and going stark white. I sympathized, and tried to change her mind, but Shinobu just kept repeating, "I'll do it."

Finally she looked at me with tears in her eyes and asked, "You don't want me to do it, Keitaro?"

What could I do?

I finally understood why Naru tried to check me out, yet seemed disgusted by the very idea. She was trying to spare the other girls from having to look at me.

"I see," I murmured. I stood up to go.

Shinobu hastily tugged on the hem of my pants, and since my belt was loose, my pants slipped down to my ankles just like that. Shinobu was so shocked, she fell face-first onto the tatami mat. "Ow!"

"Are you all right, Shinobu?"

"Yes. But where are you going, Keitaro?"

Normally, I wouldn't leave a damsel in distress behind, but I had to get out of there. I'll be the first to admit it—I'm a wimp. "I'm such a fool. I can't do this with just anyone. I'm sorry."

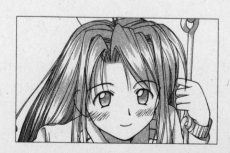

Somehow, I ended up going to Naru's room. She didn't even look up when I entered. I sat on the other side of her desk, wondering how to strike up a conversation.

Naru looked like she could care less if I stayed, or curled up and died on the floor. She simply continued to write furiously in her notebook. The only sound in the room was the scratching of her pencil.

"Well," I began. "I really don't get girls."

Naru remained silent, scratching away.

I continued, "Why were you mad about Kitsune? And why was Motoko mad about you and I . . . ? Maybe the reason was . . ."

Underneath the desk, my leg accidentally brushed against Naru's—it felt soft and silky and I got so distracted that I stopped in mid-sentence. I thought she'd give me a Naru Kick or a Naru Punch, but she didn't do a thing.

Maybe she just didn't notice we were touching.

But her pencil stilled. Her hands didn't move. We both sat there, frozen.

Finally she pulled her legs back and said, "What?"

"What 'what?' " I asked, confused.

"Maybe the reason was what?"

Oh, she was asking me to finish my sentence. I don't even really remember what I was talking about. I just didn't have the right words to ask why the Hinata House girls seemed to hate me, but acted a little jealous over me. I figured I'd skip it and just jump to the point.

"Can you look?"

"At what?" she asked.

"The treasure map."

Naru threw her pencil at my head. "What a dope!"

I sighed. "Yep. I'm a dope."

"You didn't want me to do it when I tried!"

"I know. I still don't want you to," I said.

She shrugged. "So just quit the whole thing."

I cleared my throat. "I don't want to show my body to anyone, not even you."

Naru looked hurt. She bit her lip.

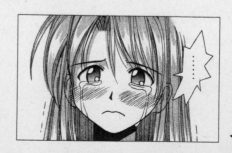

"But," I quickly said, "if I *had* to show it to someone, you are the only person that comes to mind, Narusegawa. I can only imagine it would be you. No one else."

Naru stood up and yelled, enraged, "What do you mean, 'imagine it would be me?' You're telling me you fantasize about me checking you out? Pervert!"

"That's n-n-not what I meant!" I stammered.

"Oh really?" She stomped her foot.

I just shook my head and sat there, looking stupid. I'm no good with words, and when talking to Naru, it always turns into a disaster.

She stared down at me coldly, then sighed and threw up her hands in exasperation. "Strip! Let's just get this ridiculous thing over with so I can get back to my studies!"

I'd actually pictured *Naru* taking my clothes off, but I knew better than to say that out loud. I didn't have a death wish.

This was weird.

I'd been checked over by Kitsune twice, and Suu and Sara that one time in my sleep. Naru did all the same things they'd done. But unlike Kitsune's sexually

aggressive style, or Suu and Sara's painful explorations, Naru stayed extremely calm and gentle. Her feather-light touches titillated me, and I struggled to contain my excitement.

I stripped and lay down on the table. Naru checked me over inch by inch. My whole body tingled. The fact that I was naked and she wasn't kinda sparked the situation even more. Several times I had to resist the urge to embrace her.

Naru was strictly professional about the whole thing. I'd hoped she didn't want the other girls to see my body because she secretly felt possessive of me. But the more objectively Naru conducted her search, the more I realized that was just a hopeless fantasy.

Maybe she's really just after the treasure. Maybe she just wants it for herself and was mad at the other girls looking at me because she didn't want to share!

It didn't really matter to me. I was in heaven with her so close to me, and the pleasurable sensations of

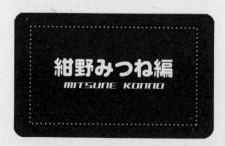

紺野みつね編
MITSUNE KONNO

her touch dulled any anger or shock I might have had. If anyone was going to discover the treasure, I'd want it to be Naru.

I didn't get girls. I don't think I ever will. But if treasure would make Naru happy, then I'd be happy too.

"There. Isn't this it?" Naru asked. She pointed at something between my shoulder blades. I couldn't quite reach it.

"There are a few bumps here," she said. "It looks like the layout of the Hinata House complex."

"Really?"

"Here's the south building, here's the north one . . . and this large bump between those two—isn't it the old annex?"

I pictured the Hinata House grounds in my mind. Naru was talking about the small additional building that was situated in the gap that was shaped like a "V." The annex had been boarded up ever since I was a child.

"There? But it's dangerous. Grandma said never to enter it. The floors are probably rotten . . ."

BAM! BOOM!

A dull pain bloomed at the back of my head and then I passed out.

I don't know how long I was unconscious, and I didn't bother looking at my watch. I ran out of Naru's room, cut through the inner lawn, and raced past the pond and to the old annex.

The wooden panels that normally covered the entrance had been peeled off, and the dusty foyer had footprints leading inside. I fainted again.

Shinobu eventually shook me awake. "Naru is gone," she said.

I felt a large, gnarly bump on the back of my head. Naru must have whacked me with one of her big, thick schoolbooks.

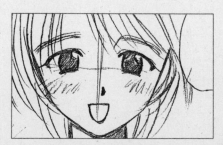

"I wonder if Narusegawa wanted the treasure badly enough to kill me?" I joked, rubbing my aching head. I never thought Naru would actually knock me out.

I told Shinobu my story and she reluctantly looked at my back (her cheeks blazing all the while, of course.)

She tilted her head. "Keitaro, I think this is just a heat rash."

"Huh?"

She handed me her compact mirror. I twisted around and peeked—sure enough, there were a bunch of little hives just under my shoulder blades. But . . . Naru had said the bumps looked like the layout of the Hinata House . . . I guess that's just what she *wanted* to see.

Besides, Grandma could do a lot of irritating things to me, but she couldn't give me a permanent heat rash.

Nevertheless, Naru must have thought she'd found the true map.

The sun started to set. There wasn't any more time for idle speculation. If I didn't get to Naru soon, she'd be stuck in that dangerous building, lost with no lights.

I started toward the annex when Shinobu said, "I'm going too."

"Oh, no you're not," I insisted. "If I don't come out soon, you have to go get help."

Shinobu looked disappointed, but nodded.

As I expected, the annex smelled like earth and wet, nasty mold. The hallway was dark and eerie, practically buried in dirt.

"Naru? Hey, Narusegawa!" I called out. "Are you there? It's really dangerous in here!" There was no answer.

I searched every room on the first floor. They were all built Western-style and it reminded me of an old European hotel.

I didn't see hide nor hair of Naru.

"Narusegawa!" I hollered as loud as I could.

SHOOM! SMASH!

The chandelier came crashing down, slightly grazing my side. I squinted up at the ceiling. The fastenings must have rusted over time and just couldn't support its weight.

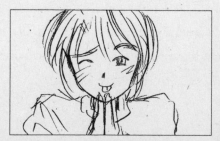

This place was honestly dangerous. I quickly dashed back to the foyer. Then I noticed an obscure set of stairs behind a thick column. It had to have been the back steps for employees.

As I climbed the staircase, I heard a faint giggle. It totally creeped me out. This place was an ideal horror movie set, I swear.

"Na-Narusegawa?" I tried to sound manly, but it came out in an embarrassing squeak.

The giggling suddenly stopped.

Then I heard Naru. "Keitaro, you are such a dope!"

I ran up the stairs. Naru was in the room on the right. She looked down at the floor, where dozens of papers were strewn and scattered around her feet.

She laughed so hard, she looked possessed. I couldn't keep my eyes off her. I'd never seen her giggle so much.

"A real dope," she said, pointing at me.

"Ah, yeah . . . I guess I'm not all that smart, but . . ."

"Keitaro Urashima!" Naru said happily, her voice echoing strangely. "Third grade, second quarter, science test score—twenty-three points!"

"What? What's that?" I asked, stepping forward.

Naru ignored me and picked up another sheet of paper. "Third grade, first quarter, math test score—thirty points."

She picked up another. "Second grade, second quarter, literature—twenty-five points!"

I picked up one of the stray papers. At the top was my childish handwriting: *Keitaro Urashima.* There were about a bazillion red marks and a devastatingly low score emblazoned on the bottom.

Naru cupped her cheek and tried to stop laughing. "These are all your old test forms. You sure had terrible grades, even as early as elementary school!"

"Not all of them," I protested. "I just hid the really bad ones . . . But what are they all doing here—ah ha!"

I remembered. During my elementary school years, I had a bunch of bad grades I didn't want my parents to see. I used to hide them in my desk drawer, but I was afraid my folks would find them. So one winter when I

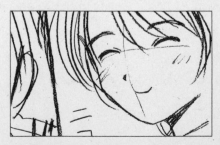

visited Grandma, I showed them to her, and asked her to keep them secret.

Grandma had smiled and said she'd hide my precious things in a safe place.

I never expected that she'd put them *here,* though.

"So, this was the treasure?" Naru asked. " 'Keitaro's secret, important thing?' "

I nodded. "When Grandma called, it was probably about these. She probably wanted Aunt Haruka to get them out of the rubble, since this place is falling apart."

It still didn't make sense though—Naru figured out coming here just by looking at my totally random heat rash. It was like . . . fate.

"Maybe it was just dumb luck," Naru suggested.

"Lucky or not, we finally found the treasure."

Naru chuckled as she picked up all the papers.

I was relieved, but a little disappointed. It was like finding out Moby Dick was really a goldfish or something. All that hype for nothing. "Maybe we shouldn't show these to Kitsune. She'll probably flip her lid."

I imagined I'd have to wait on her hand and foot until she forgave me.

"Or Shinobu," Naru said. "She'll be crushed if she learns you were such a bad student."

I could just see Shinobu struggling to hold back her tears when she heard.

"What should I do with these?" Naru teased, holding the papers just out of reach. "Think I should just show all the girls?"

"Give them back," I demanded, reaching for them.

"No way," Naru said playfully, snatching them away. She hid them behind her back. "I found them. If you want them back, you'll have to pay. Or else, every time you do something perverted, I'll show everyone one of these!"

"I won't do anything perverted!"

"You peep at us in the bathtub."

I blanched. "Not much . . ."

"You've actually jumped in the women's bath!"

"That wasn't my fault!" I insisted.

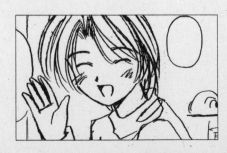

"If something like that happens again, I'll post one of these tests up at the front entrance!"

I looked closely at Naru. She was smiling, but I could tell she was kinda upset that this whole mess had been over something so silly. It wouldn't take much to make her vengeful, I figured.

"Please, give them back," I pleaded.

"Not on your life! Stay back!" She sidled away, scooping up bunches of papers.

"They belonged to me!"

"They're mine now!"

"Give them back!" I lunged forward to grab my tests, but I accidentally grabbed Naru's breast instead . . . It felt like I was squeezing a soft marshmallow.

Naru's face turned fire-engine red.

"Pervert!" she bellowed.

Just as she was about to attack me, the floor beneath us cracked and split. Naru fell flat on her rear. She pulled me down with her, and I landed with my hands full of primo-Naru-booby.

"Narusegawa, are you hurt?"

She groaned. "I twisted my ankle . . . Hey! How much longer are you gonna grope me?"

I realized I was still fondling her breasts. Normally, I would have let go and headed for the hills, but I didn't want to today. I wanted to stay close like this for a little longer, touch her some more . . .

"Na-Narusegawa . . . I'm sorry," I whispered. I still didn't let go.

"So shove off already!" she demanded, pushing me away.

We sat up. I blushed. "I meant, I'm sorry that this wasn't the treasure you were hoping for."

Naru looked at me like she was really peeved. "Did you really think I was just after some stupid treasure?"

I fidgeted. "Ah, well . . ." She had checked me over so seriously—and even bonked me on the head to knock me out, just to get to the treasure.

"You think I'm that kind of girl? You'd think I'd strip you naked just for a fortune?" She glared at me. "I'm glad

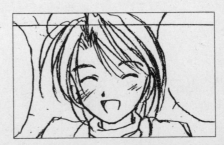

the only thing here are these stupid papers! That way, you can't leave!"

I blinked, totally confused. "I was going somewhere?"

"I heard you talking with Kitsune in the bathroom. If you guys had found a fortune, you were going to run away together, remember?"

"Naru," I countered, "a man being smothered by giant breasts is liable to agree to any crazy scheme!"

Naru looked furious. "Maybe you were just playing around, but the only reason you're staying at the Hinata House is because you're broke, right, Keitaro?"

I shrugged. "Yeah."

"So, it stands to reason that if you found a large amount of money, you could live anywhere else you wanted, right?"

"Uh, sure, but . . ." I was totally flummoxed.

"Ah! Who cares?! Stay here or not, no great loss!" She threw the papers high up in the air. They fell to the floor like little white clouds. "But it would be really tough on us girls without a manager, and Suu and Shinobu would actually miss you, and . . ."

I was such a dope. This whole time, I'd had no clue. Naru wanted me to stay.

"Narusegawa. The reason I stay here isn't because I'm poor. It's because . . ."

"Yeah?"

My heart pounded in my ears. I moved closer to her. Her lips were slightly parted, and her eyes sparkled, and she smelled like cherry blossoms. If you could forget the dark, wet, moldy surroundings, the mood was pretty romantic.

Naru's eyelashes fluttered. Swallowing I moved closer. "I stay because of y—"

Just then, the ceiling crashed in around us. Of course.

Sara whooped as the Mecha Tama (Suu's flying turtle machine) broke through the roof and crash-landed into the second-story floor. Motoko, Suu, Shinobu, and Sara all rode on its giant metallic back.

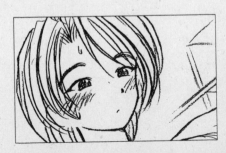

"Hey, you guys, get out of the way, will ya?" Suu shouted.

But it was too late. The mechanical turtle pulled Naru and I along as it crashed through two floors and finally burrowed deep into the basement.

The machine wheezed and then finally broke. We were all trapped inside the hole it had created when it landed. We couldn't budge the machine an inch, and if we moved around, the walls could crumble down around us at any moment.

"Thanks," Naru murmured. "What the hell were you doing?"

"Motoko said we had to hurry," Kitsune explained. "So we may have been a little careless."

"I said 'hurry.' I didn't say to barge in on the back of a giant turtle!" Motoko insisted.

"Oh dear," Shinobu said. "Look. The sun is already down."

I looked up. It was going to be a very long, dark, hot summer night.

Most people would probably consider this a crisis. But this is just normal for the Hinata House.

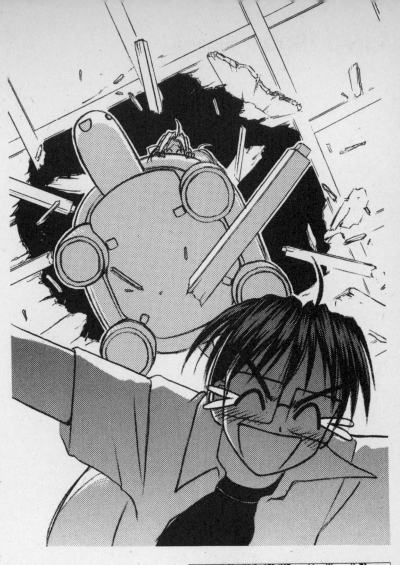
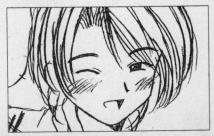

I usually would have panicked, but I was too preoccupied.

Naru was pressed up against me. We both squeezed together in the small space, our limbs entangled. I noticed that Naru pointedly hid my test papers behind her back, so the other girls wouldn't see.

Why is Naru keeping my secret? I wondered.

If I believed what she'd said, then Naru probably wanted to find the treasure before I did and hide it to prevent me from leaving. She'd threatened to use the test papers against me, but now she was keeping them safe.

In my whole life, I'd never had a girl care about me, or do something nice for me. It was hard for me to trust Naru. After all, I didn't get girls. This was probably just another one of my dumb fantasies.

But I kinda wanted to believe it. If it were true, if Naru really did care for me, then, I'd be really happy.

I don't get girls. But I still keep hoping . . .

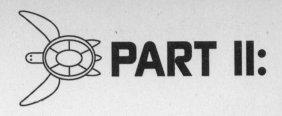

PART II:

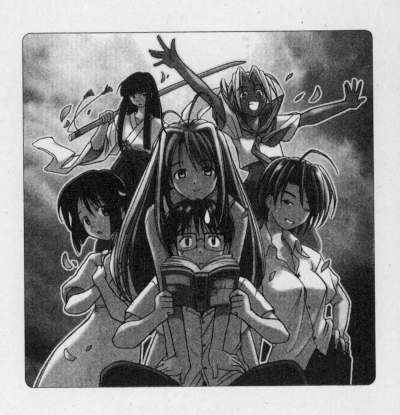

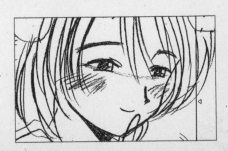

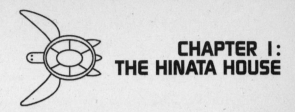

CHAPTER 1:
THE HINATA HOUSE

When I was little, the Hinata House was called the Hinata Inn. It used to be a little tiny lodge. I played there often as a child.

Since my family ran a store year-round, they couldn't take me on trips during summer vacations, so they just sent me to the Hinata Inn. Grandma was the manager. Now, she's traveling around the world, but back then, she stood at the front counter as if she'd been planted there, welcoming new guests.

The Hinata Inn's teashop used to be managed by Grandma's eldest daughter, Aunt Yoko. (Aunt Yoko was my mom's older sister.)

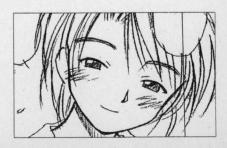

Aunt Yoko's daughter, my Aunt Haruka, came back to run the teashop after she finished with college. (Technically, Haruka and I are cousins, but because she seemed so much older than me, I started calling her "Auntie" when I was little, and it just sort of stuck.) In my family, older relatives all get nicknamed "Uncle" or "Auntie" and that's that.

Of course, every time I called Aunt Haruka "Auntie," she'd box my ears and tell me to shut up. As a child, I didn't understand, so I kept repeating the same mistake over and over, until Aunt Haruka just gave up.

You know, now that I look back, even though I sucked at gym and wasn't especially strong, I took enough beatings (especially since I've agreed to manage the Hinata House, what with Motoko's sword skills, Suu's weird inventions, Sara's full-body tackles, and Naru's punches) that nowadays, no matter how many deathblows I receive, I still manage to avoid hospitals. I'm tough mostly because Aunt Haruka beat me to a pulp for so many years.

When Aunt Haruka returned to open the teashop again, Grandma Hinata recorded her into the family registry as her adopted daughter. So, based on the

official registry, as the grandson of Grandma Hinata, I technically could call Haruka my aunt. But every time I say "Auntie," she yanks my cheeks apart or elbows me in the face.

Boy, I've really gotten off track here. My point was, back when the Hinata House used to be called the Hinata Inn, I remember Grandma yelling at me anytime I got near the annex or the pond.

At that time, there were three buildings strictly off limits to me. One was the teashop. The other was the old tower with the dangerous walkway. And finally, the annex itself. It was a small, two-story building with Western-style architecture—stained glass windows, a weathervane, slanted roofs—it was just really unique. It reminded me of the kind of mansions you'd see in movies or read about in novels. In later years, as it got more run down, it looked like a haunted house. But when I was growing up, the

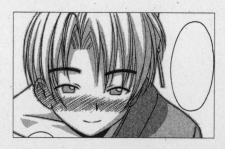

annex simply beckoned a young child like me to go exploring.

One day, I got bored. My four-year-old heart yearned for adventure. I sang the theme song to the TV show *Liddo,* and marched straight to the annex. Back then, it was just an abandoned building. It wasn't covered in rubble or mold. When I ventured into the foyer, I recall it being kinda new-looking and rather clean. It looked like somebody actually lived there.

On the first floor, at the far end of the hallway, a door was slightly ajar.

I peeked in, but someone from behind me called out, "Stop!"

Grandma grabbed me by the shoulders and dragged me out. It was a long time ago; I couldn't remember what it was that I'd seen.

Grandma Hinata took me to her room on the second floor of the south building and warned me, "Don't ever go in the annex, because it's dangerous!" Her eyes burned intensely—more so than if she had been angry. It left a really strong impression on me.

I distinctly remember calling out for Auntie Haruka, but I don't know why. Maybe my memories were starting to surface because I'd so recently gone into the annex with Naru—I have a really hard time remembering much from my childhood.

But beyond that, something else was bothering me.

I felt like . . . like whenever I was in the annex . . . I wasn't *alone*.

The Hinata House had countless fairy tales attached to it. There's a legend that if a couple stays overnight in the tower, they'll get married and live happily ever after. In the main building, there are dozens of secret passageways that connect to unknown places. Plus, Grandma collected occult trinkets as a hobby. So, the whole place had kinda a weird aura to it.

Plus, the old inn used to host annual events like cherry blossom viewing parties, and stewed sweet potato cookouts. Some of the guests Grandma told me about

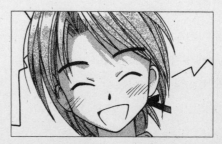

were pretty strange. And all the girls who resided here now, at the Hinata House, had peculiar quirks and odd histories.

Of course, the biggest mystery was the annex. Grandma would never give me a straight answer, and Aunt Haruka never wanted to talk about it either.

Don't get me wrong. Despite the weird aura, I never thought the Hinata House was a strange place. After all, it's home.

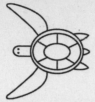

CHAPTER 2:
OPERATION: HOSPITALITY!

"**S**o, that's basically it, Keitaro. It's all yours."

Aunt Haruka handed me a notebook. I read her handwriting: *September 12th, 4 people, 2 nights. September 13th, 1 person, 1 night.* Lots of other little details were written in the margins.

I had no clue what any of this meant.

"What's this? Your vacation plan?" I asked.

She glared at me, her cigarette dangling from her lips. "They're inn customers. They'll be staying here for a few nights." She flicked her ashes away. "Grandma asked me to take care of them, but I can't just leave the shop unattended."

"Inn? Customers? Where exactly are they supposed to be staying?" I asked, disbelieving.

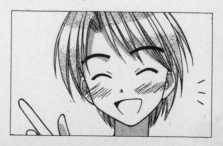

"At the Hinata House, of course."

I held my head in my hands. The Hinata House is a dormitory. I had my hands full just trying to keep things running smoothly with a couple of wacky girls; I really couldn't imagine taking care of guests.

Haruka, are you crazy?

But she wasn't kidding. She towered over me and said, "Look. You are a pathetic, three-time entrance exam loser. You're going to cram school, and you're the manager of an all-girls dorm."

"Please don't remind me."

"Just shut up and listen," she snapped. "When Grandma decided to make this place a dorm, several inn customers were saddened by this. They thought the place was really nostalgic. Grandma tried to recommend a few nearby hot springs' hotels, but they'd been coming to Hinata Inn for years, and they prefer to keep coming here . . ."

So it appeared that Grandma appeased her regular customers by promising to open the Hinata Inn once in a while, to take them in. This autumn, it was to open for four days.

"So, don't we need to call Grandma Hinata and have her come back for a week?"

"A woman's feelings are complex, Keitaro."

"What do you mean?"

Aunt Haruka sighed. "Most of the customers will be retired folks. Some of them have even been coming here since before the war."

"So?"

"So how old do you think Grandma was back then?"

I shrugged. "Um . . . Let's see . . . How old are you, Auntie?"

She slapped me on both cheeks and continued on as if I hadn't spoken. "Back then, Grandma Hinata used to be the town beauty. She attracted customers to the inn."

I couldn't imagine Grandma Hinata without tons of wrinkles. When I tried hard to picture the town beauty,

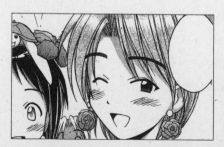

I kept seeing Naru in a silk kimono, during New Year celebrations. "I'm having a hard time believing it."

Aunt Haruka just shrugged. "Everyone was young once. Anyway, in order not to crush the regular customers' dreams, Grandma decided she'd stay away on her vacation. She doesn't want them to see her looking old. But some of these guests . . . well, they made their reservations ages ago. We can't refuse them now. We need to run Hinata Inn without Grandma, okay? So, good luck!"

Dude! There's no way I could run the Hinata Inn, even for a few days. I tried to protest, but Aunt Haruka just barreled past me, saying, "I turned in the paperwork to the city office. I got you a culinary license, so there shouldn't be any problems!"

"Paperwork is not the point!" I said. "How many customers are coming?"

"About thirty," she said nonchalantly.

I flipped out. "How can I take care of all those people all by myself?"

"I didn't say you had to do it alone, Keitaro." She lit up another cigarette, smiled, and pointed at the Hinata House. "You have a good group of employees right there."

"I'll help! I'll help!" Suu shouted, bouncing around. "You serve the guests food and alcohol, and then sleep with them, just like the geisha in the old samurai movies, right? I saw one on TV!"

I pressed the bridge of my nose between my fingers.

"Suu, don't learn weird stuff from TV!" Shinobu said, then looked at me. "Um, Keitaro . . . I think I can help with the cooking."

Shinobu was always so sweet. "Thank you," I said.

"I'll help!" Suu said again. "And Sara too!"

"Don't volunteer me," Sara said.

I sighed. "Thank you, Suu. But Sara is still in grade school, so, I can't make her work."

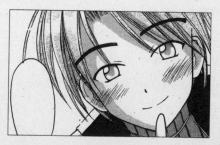

"Oh, it's all right!" Suu insisted, clutching Sara close. "This new invention of mine is a growth tonic. The blue pills make you age, and the red pills turn you back into a kid. So, no worries about those pesky child labor laws! Come on, Sara, take . . . Wait . . ." She frowned. "Was it the blue pill that made you grow? Or the red? Oh well, just try one and see."

Sara paled and tried to escape, but Suu held her close, attempting to pour the pills right into Sara's mouth.

Shinobu's eyes glazed over. "Oh dear, if only I could become a grownup too."

Suddenly, Kitsune bounced down the stairs and plucked the bottle right out of Suu's hands. "Hey, quit it."

"Aw, but . . ." Suu whined.

Kitsune interrupted her, saying, "I'll help too, Keitaro. I'm more useful than Sara, anyway."

"Quit acting so high and mighty, Kitsune!" Sara said, pouting.

I couldn't believe my ears. "Kitsune? You're actually going to *work*?"

"Yeah. Is that a problem?"

"But, Kitsune," I said, "you like naps, and drinking, and gambling. You've never had a real job. You barely graduated high school and your favorite phrase is, 'marry wealthy.' So, working at the inn might be a bit too rough for you—"

"You didn't have to go that far," Kitsune muttered. "Look. I'm a Hinata House resident. I've been here the longest, in fact. I remember when this place used to be the Hinata Inn. I'll be glad to pitch in." She gathered up her hair. "And offer . . ." she unbuttoned her blouse to expose more cleavage. " . . . my services." She licked her lips. "You doubt my sincerity, Keitaro?"

She grabbed my head and pushed my face right into her cleavage. I couldn't see a thing, but sweet softness surrounded me.

"What are you ffmmmm Kitsuneeee."

"Oh, Keitaro, if you breathe so hard like that, it's going to drive me wild!" she said in a lusty voice, and hugged me closer.

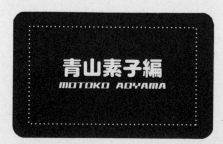

青山素子編
MOTOKO AOYAMA

"Hey, Keitaro! You'll let me work, right? Please say yes!" Sara started begging.

I almost lost my mind, right then.

Suddenly, a voice called out. "Enough already!"

KICK!

My spine almost cracked in half under the blow. Kitsune and I fell to the floor together.

"Whoa!" I yelped. Suddenly I couldn't breathe— my mouth was full of something soft. It felt . . . kinda good.

"Keitaro is sucking Kitsune's boob!" Sara squealed.

I snapped back like a spring.

"You went too far," Kitsune said darkly.

"You jerk!" Naru said, approaching me with her fists clenched. I could see flames in her eyes.

I thought it best to beg for my life. "No, Narusegawa! It was totally an accident! You're the one who kicked me . . . *Ack!*"

Naru kicked me in the mouth. She continued to stomp on my face like she was squishing the life out of a cockroach. My head slammed back onto the floor and I saw stars.

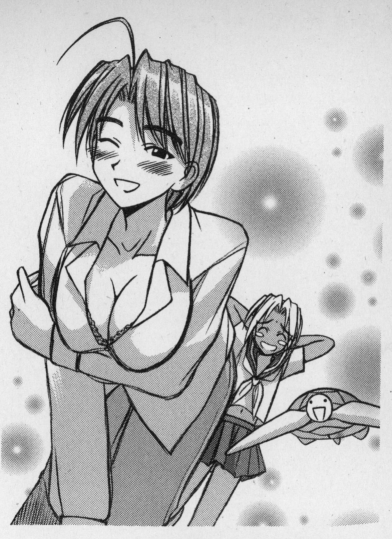
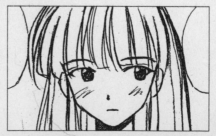

"Get it together," Naru said, glaring down at me. "You have less than a week before the customers come, right?"

I looked up, surprised. "Naru? Are you going to help me?"

"What? You don't want me to?"

"No, that's great." I expected Naru to be too busy studying to help out.

She nodded. "Your grandmother promised them, right?"

"Yes."

"Maybe some of the guests had a crush on her when she was younger."

"Grandma was married!"

"I'm talking about before that!" Naru said. "Who knows? Maybe she was in love with one special customer, but he was drafted. He came to the inn to say goodbye for the last time, but neither of them could express their true feelings!" Her eyes twinkled.

"Yeah, that's gotta be it," I said, rolling my eyes.

"But after the war, he never returned. Grandmother, in order to keep the inn in business, was forced to marry some rich guy."

Wait, wait. Rich guy? Forced to marry? So my mom and Aunt Yoko were products of a loveless marriage?

"Um . . ."

"Then one day, he was finally released from a POW camp in Siberia. He traveled all the way back here, and stood before the inn, anxious to see his one true love." She sighed. "But life is cruel. Grandmother was married, with children. They didn't speak a word, but only gazed into each other's eyes and wondered what might have been."

Naru stepped closer, straddling me. "Grandmother stepped toward him, but she couldn't speak. She couldn't keep her promise, so instead she remained behind, and turned the inn into an all-girls dormitory."

"Um, that was a pretty recent development," I reminded her.

"Oh, that's right." Naru snapped out of her fantasy. She scratched her head. "But, you don't know. Maybe

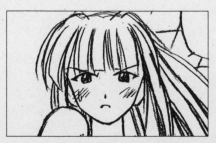

there was some kind of romantic promise, and that's why Grandmother won't come back from her trip—she can't bear to face him. Oh! These kind of stories make me swoon!" She sighed. "That's why I'll help you, Keitaro."

I looked up at Naru's sweet face, but along the way, my eyes sort of got sidetracked by her silky legs, her little plaid skirt, and the tantalizing view of her tiny, white panties.

My brain fried.

POW!

Naru jumped up and pulled her legs together. Her feet landed right on my crotch. It was the kind of move that would have made a pro-wrestler proud. It crushed my manhood like a worm in a winepress, let me tell you.

I couldn't even make a sound. I just squirmed around, tears streaming down my face.

Naru grabbed me up by the collar and screamed, "I was talking about a good story and you were staring up my skirt!"

"You're the one that showed—!"

"Showed? Me? Why would I show that to you? You dirty pig!"

I couldn't move. I knew she was going to punch me into the stratosphere, but I was paralyzed with pain and fear.

Suddenly, someone screamed, a shrill feminine voice that cut through the inner lawn of the Hinata House.

We ran toward the scream. When we arrived, we found Motoko lying unconscious on the inner lawn.

She was wearing a pure white *hakama,* her samurai kimono. She had a white headband around her forehead, and Shisui in her hands. (Normally she practiced her *katas* with a sword replica; I had to be careful when I moved Shisui or I'd cut my fingers off.)

"What's wrong, Motoko?" I whispered as she blinked awake.

"Uh . . . ah . . ." Slowly, she opened her eyes. Suddenly, Tama the hot springs turtle waddled out of the folds of her kimono.

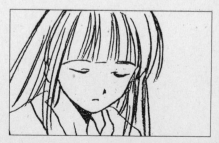

Motoko writhed. "Get it, get it, get it! Urashima, get it!" She broke out into a cold sweat and clung to me.

"How am I supposed to . . . ?"

Even as we spoke, Tama crawled back into the folds of Motoko's kimono.

"Ah! Stop! Please! Get it, get it, *please!*" She clung tighter to me, panting slightly. Her hands tightened on my shoulders, and her eyes glistened with tears.

I knew she hated turtles, and she was really upset right then. I wanted to remove Tama, but at that moment, she was squirming and clinging so much, I couldn't really move my hands. In order to get Tama out, I'd have to touch Motoko's breasts, and frankly, I'm stupid, but not *that* stupid.

But Motoko was seriously starting to freak, so I reached my hand in and . . .

"What a lame excuse to grope a girl!" Naru said, disgusted. She pulled me away from Motoko and threw me in the pond.

"Why me?" I whined.

"Myu-myu," Tama squeaked. He jumped out of Motoko's kimono and, as only Tama could, flew toward the Hinata House.

Motoko was still in shock. Her chest heaved as she took gasping breaths. It was kind of adorable. When she finally got herself under control, she insisted, "I didn't scream because of that stupid turtle! I'm used to living with that thing by now, you know."

She really can be adorable.

"Sure, Motoko," I said, nodding.

"No, I mean it. I screamed because of what I sensed."

We all stared at her. "What do you mean?" Naru asked.

"Just recently, you and Urashima were drawn to the annex . . ."

I tried to explain that I had actually just followed Naru to the annex, and she wasn't drawn there, she

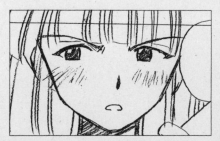

decided to go there because of my stupid heat rash, but Motoko just plowed on.

"We went there to save Naru," she said.

I wanted to remind her that they actually barged in on a giant Mecha Tama, but Motoko was on a roll.

"And the moment we stepped foot inside, it felt . . . familiar. Nostalgic."

She looked far away, then continued. "After a few days, I was able to figure out why it felt so familiar. It's very similar to the *jiryoudo* at my house."

"Jiryou . . . do?" Shinobu asked.

"Is that some kinda food?" Suu asked.

Motoko remained serious. "It's a spirit-containment temple," she clarified. "You all know that my family uses the traditional secret sword skills of the shin mei ryu. The most skilled swordsman in my family traditionally undertakes the responsibility of exorcising bad ghosts— you know, demons and evil spirits and the like." She searched the girls' faces. "You don't believe me?"

Sara blushed. "It's so unscientific."

Motoko coughed, choosing to ignore that line of reasoning. "Some evil spirits wouldn't perish, so we had

no choice but to contain them. Over the generations, the temple became a place to imprison evil spirits. We called it the jiryoudo."

I nodded, like I had any clue what the heck she was talking about. Bottom line: the annex had the same feeling as a prison for bad ghosts.

Everyone gulped.

Shinobu covered her ears and shifted her weight uncomfortably.

"I had to wonder why the annex felt the same as the temple," Motoko said. "To tell you the truth, I felt a strong spiritual power from Grandma Hinata. I'm not sure of the details, but I believe the shin mei ryu ancestry and the Urashima family line were somehow connected in the past. It was my destiny to study martial arts at this place."

I just stared at her.

"So, maybe there was an evil spirit that the Urashima family has trapped here. Maybe it was attracted to

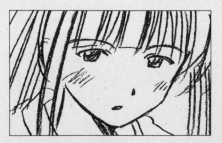

Keitaro and his amazingly bad luck. Maybe it wished to resurrect—"

"Forget it," I mumbled. "No way."

Annoyed, Motoko pointed her sword at me. "Shut up, Urashima."

I flinched. "Don't hurt me!"

Motoko sighed. "In preparation for going into the annex, I cleansed my soul, wore pure white, and brought Shisui, but . . ." She hesitated.

"What happened?" Kitsune asked, curious.

Suu was bored by the story, and had fallen asleep in Motoko's lap. Shinobu was still covering her ears. "Is it over yet?" she kept asking.

"Come on, Motoko, what happened?" Naru pressed.

"Actually . . ." Motoko swallowed. "When I opened the door, it looked different. The rubble was gone. The interior was clean and airy. As if someone were living there."

Somehow, this story sounded familiar to me.

"For a moment, I thought Shinobu had cleaned the annex," Motoko said, "but the ceiling and walls looked

brand new. That made me suspicious. I climbed the stairs and was astounded. The hole we made in the ceiling wasn't there!"

I started feeling afraid. Just last week, the Mecha Tama crashed through the ceiling, two floors, and buried itself in the basement. Haruka really laid us out because there wasn't enough money to fix the damage.

~~If this were a manga, perhaps the assistant illustrator forgot to draw the hole. If it had been an anime, maybe the scriptwriter had forgotten about last week's episode. But this was a novel . . . No, I mean, reality . . .~~

"Is it over now?" Shinobu squeaked, her hands still over her ears.

Everyone ignored her. The only sound was the clattering of Sara's teeth.

"Then, I heard a noise on the first floor," Motoko continued. "Someone was there. I quickly ran

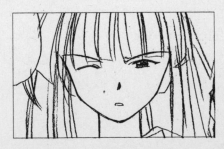

downstairs. There was something near the entrance . . . I saw someone on the other side of the door . . ."

Okay, I was ready to pee my pants.

"Or at least, that's what I sensed," Motoko told us. "But then, my vision went dark. It smelled raw and moldy. I squirmed and coughed."

Shinobu whimpered.

"What happened then, Motoko?" Kitsune urged.

"Let's just forget this story," Sara suggested. Sara was usually the first one to make a joke out of stuff like this, but now she was pale and tense.

"Everyone just calm down!" Naru said, but she looked like she was ready to bolt, too.

"Narusegawa, where do you think you're going?" I asked.

But then I realized my own feet were leading me back in the direction of the Hinata House.

"You guys," Motoko said, anguished.

"Was it Tama? Did he scare you?" Suu asked, rubbing her sleepy eyes.

Motoko's face gradually reddened and she hunched her shoulders. "Yes. My apologies."

So . . . So, Motoko hadn't seen anyone in the annex—she'd just mistaken Tama for an evil spirit.

I don't get girls.

We all headed toward the annex, but it looked exactly as we had left it. There was a hole in the ceiling, and rubble all over the floor.

Motoko looked confused. Finally, she said, "I must have hallucinated. I must redo my training from the beginning."

She went back to her room and tried to pack her things to return to the temple, but of course, we stopped her and managed to convince her to stay.

That night, Naru and I whispered through the hole that connected our rooms.

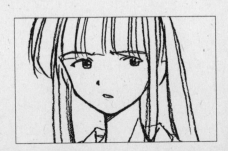

"If Motoko said she hallucinated, then that's probably what happened," Naru said.

I wondered. "Motoko has special spiritual powers, though. Maybe she did see something strange."

"Knock it off."

I couldn't see her through the hole, but I could tell just by her voice that she was a little angry. "I was there all by myself, remember? There were no creepy spirits."

I sighed. Just the thought of Naru all alone in that building, poking around dangerous places for treasure . . . it made me shiver.

"Keitaro, please don't make me think something was in there with me," she pleaded. She sounded really weirded out.

I teased her, "Who-o-o-o-o kno-o-o-o-ws? Maybe something creepy followed you back and is going to watch you while you sleep!"

There was no answer. Was she too scared to speak? Maybe she'd be too afraid to sleep by herself, and she'd jump down through the hole, and cuddle up to me for the rest of the night. (Hey, a guy can dream, right?) I kept waiting for her to say something.

I didn't like the strange silence.

To tell you the truth, I couldn't just brush off Motoko's story. I don't really remember everything clearly, but I had a similar experience. When I wandered into the annex as a small child, the interior was pristine. Even then, it was an abandoned building. But it was tidy. And I met someone. I don't remember her face, but I do remember it was a woman.

I paced my room, trying to recall that lady's face. I drew back my curtain and stared out at the old annex.

What if I saw that woman in there?

Okay, I was wigging out.

Instead of worrying about the annex, I should have been worrying about Naru. *I'm not really afraid, but if little things bother me, Naru must be freaking out. She's been so quiet. Maybe she's waiting for me to come to her. Gosh, she's so adorable. If she wants me to take care of her, I guess I'll have to . . .*

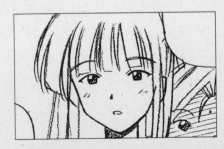

I stacked a bunch of books together, used them as a stepladder, and pulled myself up through the hole. "Hey, Narusegawa?"

I saw her wriggling on the floor, her loose robe almost completely open. She was tangled up in a kimono. Her thighs, chest, belly . . . practically everything was exposed. Only tiny scraps of cloth covered her intimate parts.

I gotta tell you, this was way sexier than seeing her totally nude.

Most of the kimono bunched up at her feet, and somehow her *obi* belt was wrapped several times around her slender waist, down around her thighs, and up over her bulging breasts. She looked like she'd been tied up. It was really erotic.

Naru struggled to remove the *obi*. She glared at me. "What the hell are you looking at?!"

CRASH! RUMBLE!

Naru Body Tackle! I tumbled headfirst back down into my room.

"Don't just peek in a girl's room like that!" she yelled through the hole.

"I'm sorry! I had no idea what you were doing!" I said. "I thought you were in danger!"

"Danger? What do you mean?" She peered through the hole. "Quit blushing. You better not be having some weird fantasy!"

I noticed Naru was blushing, herself.

"I was just trying to practice wearing the hot springs kimono."

I laughed. "It looked like the kimono was wearing *you*. Why don't you just have Aunt Haruka help you?"

She huffed. "It's embarrassing for a girl not to know how to wear a kimono," Naru confessed. "I'll have to wear it every day next week, so . . ."

I smiled. The younger girls offered to help, and Kitsune too. Motoko said helping out was the least she could do after the annex incident. Aunt Haruka had agreed to take care of Sara while she minded the teashop. And now, with Naru at my side, I knew next week would go well.

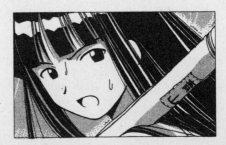

Only one problem remained. I needed to study like mad before the guests came. Sigh.

"It's delicious!" I blurted out.

Shinobu looked down and covered her blushing cheeks with her hands. She looked so happy. "Thank you, Keitaro."

I poked my chopsticks at all the little dishes of food laid out on the cafeteria table. Shinobu had made all sorts of things to serve the inn customers. Each delicacy tasted great, like home-cooked meals.

"Food was my biggest concern, but now, there's no problem!" I said. "When we open, Naru and I will help you cook and serve the guests. I'm sorry you have to wake up early in the morning to make breakfast, though."

"That's okay," Shinobu said. "But, Keitaro, are you sure we don't have to move out of our rooms?" She fretted, even as she prepared the next dish.

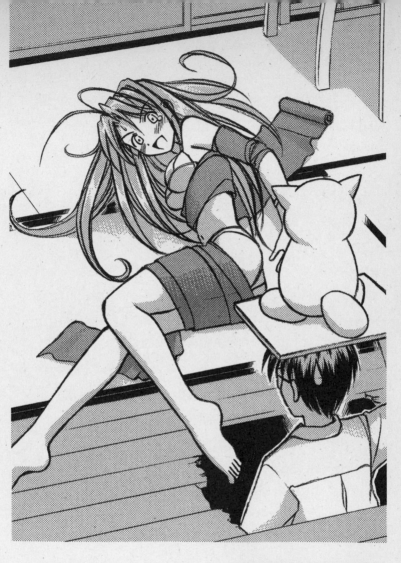
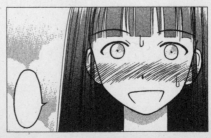

"Don't you worry," I told her. "The most we'll get is three groups in one day. We can just put everyone in the north building's vacant rooms. Besides, if we tried to clean up the south building, Suu's room alone would take about a thousand days."

Suu's room was like a tropical jungle. She had a bunch of plants and trees growing everywhere. Steam from the boiler room leaked over into her bedroom. It was practically a sauna. Cleaning up the mold and plants and all that would require a lot of effort.

"That's true," Shinobu agreed.

Suddenly, an arm popped out of nowhere. A greedy hand stole some food.

"Eeek!" Shinobu squealed.

"Suu?" I gasped. She'd climbed up next to the cutting board, and was stealing some of Shinobu's samples.

"I heard you guys mention me," she said.

"Well . . ." I trailed off.

"As punishment for your gossiping, I will confiscate Shinobu's yummy food!" She chortled. "Oooh, this heart-shaped rice ball looks good!"

She swiped the rice ball up. It was covered in pink sprinkles. It looked like it took a long time to make.

Vaguely, I wondered who Shinobu wanted to give a heart-shaped rice ball to.

"No! Suu! That's not a sample item!" Shinobu pleaded. "No, please!"

But Suu gulped it down and grinned.

Shinobu dropped to her knees weakly. "Oh dear."

"That was tasty!" Suu patted Shinobu's head. "But now it's my turn with you, Keitaro!"

She pushed me out of the cafeteria. I saw Shinobu sit there, still in shock, watching us as we left.

The women's bath and the main pool area was drastically different. Suu had planted a bunch of exotic, mysterious

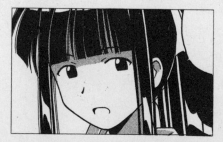

flowers and plants. There were banana and coconut trees, papaya and kiwi sprouts, etc. In addition to Tama, other tropical creatures I'd never seen before were crawling about. In the middle of one pond was a statue of a goddess.

"Do you like what I've done with the place?" Suu looked up at me with puppy dog eyes.

But I said, "Rejected!"

"Why?" she whined. "Why, why, why? It looks like a theme park! Isn't that cool?"

Suu jumped on my shoulders and wrapped her legs around my neck. She pulled my hair. (In case you were wondering, I am not, in fact, a horse, and I don't like being treated as such.)

"Suu," I said, struggling not to drop her. "All the customers are grownups. They're coming to the hot springs to relax and wash away the grime and fatigue of everyday life. A theme park isn't exactly—"

"I know all that!" Suu insisted, pulling my clothes off. She pushed me face-down into the wash area. "Keitaro, your skin is so soft," she cooed. "And you have a cute butt!"

"What?!" I cried.

"Okay, act like a customer about to receive my special services! Ready? Go!" She started to massage me. Thank God I wasn't completely naked. Look, Suu was a junior high school student. She was just innocently playing with me. But I'm a red-blooded male. It was very hard for me not to get carried away.

"Okay. We're gonna get the grime off you in no time!" Suu said. She slowly began to wriggle against me.

I've only ever seen this sort of thing in magazines and videos. It was the kind of dance girls did in certain "specialty stores." You know, where the girl uses her own body to massage and wash the guy's body?

Oh wow. It's heaven. Where did you learn this trick, Suu? I thought. *My, how you've grown . . .*

BROOOOOM BROOOOOM BROOOOOM!

I heard an engine start. Suddenly, my back felt like it was on fire. Something scraped against me—it felt like sandpaper!

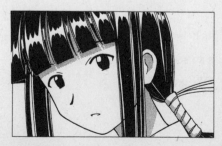

"OW! Suu, that's too rough!" I screamed.

"Does it feel good, Keitaro?" she shouted over the noise.

I glanced over my shoulder. Suu was squatting down, a maniacal grin on her face. She'd placed some sort of mechanical invention on my back.

"This is the Uki-uki Aka-suri Machine. I call it Asura!"

I squealed.

A strange robot, which had three faces and a zillion little appendages, was clinging to my back. The engine roared. Scrubber brushes attached to the appendages twirled at a super speed. This thing looked like it could take off a layer or two of *skin!*

"Help meeee!" I tried to stand up, but Asura's appendages wrapped around me and pressed me down harder. "Ugh!"

I squirmed, rolling around like a potato worm, trying to make it to the bath.

SPLOOSH! Asura and I splashed into the pool. Asura's grip loosened and I freed myself. Gasping, I clawed my way to the surface.

"A-a-achoo! I'm safe, right?"

Suddenly, something poked me, right in the crotch. "Huh? What . . . ?" It wasn't Asura. It was a fish!

Suu came to the edge of the bath and bragged, "I studied a book about fish! The bream and flatfish will dance for you!"

"Oh. The bream and flatfish are harmless, but . . . But, Suu! If you put a fish in a hot spring, it'll get cooked in no time!"

I grabbed a fish and pulled it out of the water. But then I realized, it wasn't a bream or flatfish at all. It was long, with a large mouth and shiny black eyes.

"Well," Suu said, "bream and flatfish were expensive, so I got some hot springs fish from my homeland!"

"H-h-hot springs fish?"

She nodded. "They can live in hot water. I'm sure the customers will like them. There's just one tiny problem . . ."

POKE! POKE! CHOMP! CHOOMP!

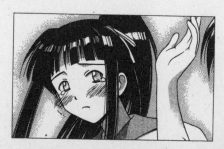

"Ow!" I pulled one of my legs out of the water—a bunch of hot springs fish were biting down on me!

"Don't tell me these little buggers are *carnivorous?!*"

"Bingo!"

"Yaaaah!" I scrambled out of the bath and checked to make sure I still had all my toes. "Freaking man-eating fish!"

Suu looked disappointed. "They're no good?"

I was about to reply, when the goddess statue wobbled from side to side, then started to slowly walk toward us.

"Awesome!" Sara said. She waved her hands out of the goddess' mouth. "How about this, Keitaro? It's the Otohime Robot! I modeled it after that turtle-girl in Okinawa!"

(This past spring, after I failed my entrance exam yet again, I took a trip to ease my grief. I met a girl named Mutsumi Otohime. She kissed me . . . but why was I thinking about all that right now?)

I was speechless. The Otohime Robot approached me. It suddenly lost its balance. I stood there as the mechanical goddess tumbled toward me.

"Wow, talk about bad luck!"

Kitsune, who was sitting next to me, roared with laughter.

I stared at the food tray in front of me. After I told Suu and Sara that they would have to clean up the bath area, I informed them that I wanted to practice my customer service, and I returned to the manager's room.

"Aw. Are you tired?" Kitsune asked. "Shall I rub your shoulders?"

"No! It's okay, really," I said quickly. After being massaged by a psychotic robot, gnawed on by hot springs' piranhas, and almost squished by a statue, I wasn't really up for any more physical contact.

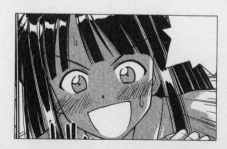

"Relax," Kitsune whispered. "Today, you're playing the role of a customer, right?"

Slowly, she massaged my shoulders. I grumbled, but it actually felt kinda good. "It's nice," I mumbled.

"Really? I hope the customers enjoy it too."

I nodded. "They will, I'm sure. But do we really want to offer massages?"

"What are you saying?" Kitsune asked, stopping cold. "A business is a business, even if it's only for four days! And most of the folks are elderly, trying to enjoy their retirement life! *Tsk, tsk!*"

Kitsune's comment made me a little uneasy, but I just concentrated on the soft sensations of her touch as she resumed massaging me.

"Please, have a drink." She poured me a glass.

"Wow. You're a pro at this."

I took a sip, but immediately spit it out. "This is real alcohol!"

"Of course. I was planning on sharing that!"

I sighed. "This is just practice, remember? What's the point of making me drink real liquor?"

"Quit worrying so much," Kitsune said. "Here, have some more." She poured another drink, then leaned close to me.

I confess I was getting aroused. In an effort to calm down, I kept drinking until my eyes started glazing over.

Kitsune was wearing the employee kimono, but the front was wide open, accenting her ample cleavage. Occasionally, I glimpsed her legs, too. It was kind of cool to see a girl in an authentic kimono.

When Kitsune noticed I was checking her out, she chuckled and took my cup away. Then she took my right hand and brought it to her left sleeve. "Did you know?" she whispered.

"What?"

"When you wear a kimono formally, you're not supposed to put on any underwear."

I gulped. "Oh really?"

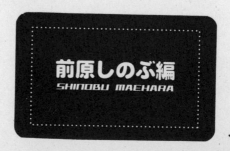

前原しのぶ編
SHINOBU MAEHARA

"You wanna check for yourself? It's pretty exciting, isn't it? To put your hand in here." She guided my right hand inside her sleeve . . . farther . . . farther . . . farther up.

"That tickles!" she said, giggling. "You need to go deeper, Keitaro. Come on, almost there."

"Ki-Kitsune . . ." I didn't know what to do, so I just wiggled my fingers. "I wonder, as your friend, if I should really continue . . . ?"

Just then, the door sliced diagonally into two halves and crumbled apart.

"Whoa!" I yelped.

Motoko and Narusegawa stood outside. Naru glared at me with dark, shining eyes. "Urashima!" she hissed. "Having yourself a blast?"

"No, it was Kitsune's idea!" I babbled.

But Kitsune had taken cover in a corner. She called out, "I told him how I was trying to earn money from the customers. I was showing him stuff worth five thousand—no—ten thousand yen!"

I looked at her like she was crazy. What the hell was she plotting? Why was she trying to make all this out to be my fault?

"Oh, we totally understand, Kitsune," Motoko said coldly, turning on me. "Urashima. I want to show you something."

I swallowed. "What's that, Motoko?" *Please not Shisui. Please not Shisui.*

"I was thinking I could please the customers," she said, drawing Shisui high over her head, "with a traditional sword dance."

"Ah . . . I t-t-think t-t-that's a little hardcore," I said.

"You will watch me perform!" Motoko commanded.

She swung the blade down, and an eerie energy aura surrounded it. I tried to run away, but Naru grabbed my arm. I hid behind her.

"Narusegawa, help!" I whispered.

"Keitaro?" she said sweetly.

"Yes?"

"Die!" she bellowed.

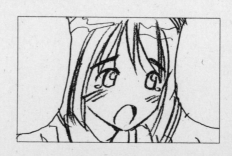

She swung me around and sent me flying straight toward Motoko. The sword swiped sideways and hurled me out the window. "Ahhhhhhh!"

As I fell back toward Earth, I wondered if I'd manage to survive until the inn opened.

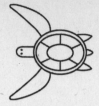

CHAPTER 3: CUSTOMERS, RUNNING AWAY!

"**T**hank you for coming! Welcome to the Hinata Inn!"

Our customers were elated. No wonder—the Hinata girls in their cute little kimonos, lined up at the tidy front entrance, were nothing short of a vision.

Naru looked so elegant in her outfit. Shinobu had put her hair up like she was undergoing her *shichi-go-san*, the celebration for third, fifth, and seventh year students. Motoko was tall and regal; her feminine frame accentuated by the kimono. Suu's tanned skin matched her kimono—she looked healthy and happy. And, of course, Kitsune looked really sexy. Even Sara had somehow slipped into the lineup . . .

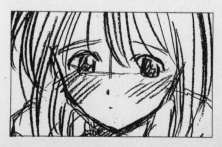

Wow. Everyone looked so grown up. I got a little choked up, like a father on his daughter's wedding day, or something. I was just brimming over with pride.

Show time!

I took the lead, and guided the customers to their rooms.

From that point on, the peace and quiet ended.

Looking back, the customers were all elderly couples, besides one group of old fellas. These people had traveled a lot; they were practically professional critics.

As the Hinata Inn supervisor, I received all sorts of complaints.

"Son, I want to change my room," one said. "The window is facing northeast."

"Can I take a bath now?" an older male customer asked.

I smiled and explained that the bath was females-only until seven o' clock, and then it was open to males-only.

"Females as in grannies, right? I won't do anything to them," he said, "so come on, now."

"I'm sorry, sir."

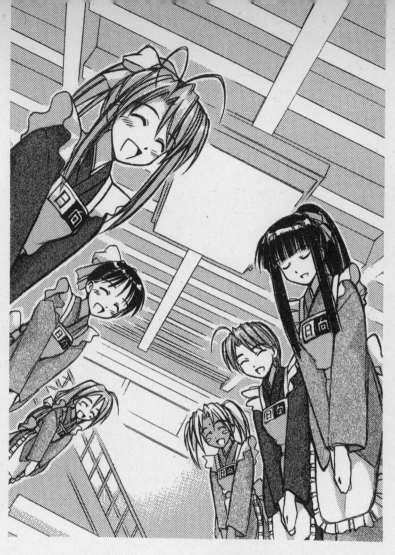

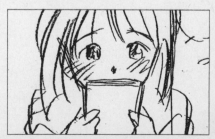

"We can do mixed bathing, can't we fellas?" he called out to his bachelor friends. They came over and tried to gang up on me, insisting they had no problems with co-ed bathing. (As if the ladies desperately wanted to bask in the glory of their wrinkly old butts.)

And that was just the beginning.

They asked us to adjust mealtimes. They asked the teashop to lower its prices. People barged into our private rooms and took pictures. Generally, the guests treated us like slaves.

Everyone kept saying how nostalgic everything was. I had to bite my tongue about a million times. They complained about the food, the hot springs temperature, the size of the rooms, the dust on the windows, and the lack of luster on the hallway floor.

I almost passed out.

Every time I climbed the stairs, I made a mental list of things to do, like retrieve extra towels, wake Mister Shibata in Room 3, take out the trash, then go buy cigarettes . . .

Suddenly, someone kicked me down the stairs. Both of us tumbled down the steps. I blinked and struggled to get my bearings.

"Narusegawa!"

"Watch where you're going!" She looked peeved. She covered me, facing away, her thighs on either side of my face. I got a nice view of her rear. Ordinarily, finding myself in this position with Naru would be a dream come true, but at the moment, I was just plain cranky. I gently pushed her off.

"You're so heavy, I can't breathe!"

"What did you say about my weight?" She tried to stand up, but fell back down on me. "Ouch!"

"Ow!" I raised my head, and accidentally peered right into the bottom opening of Naru's kimono.

Oh gosh, I need to get out of here pronto. She'll kill me!

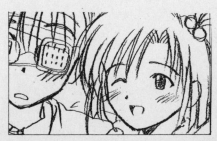

I tried not to look, but I ended up seeing—well, there wasn't the normal flash of white cotton panty that I normally saw, so that meant . . .

I jerked back. Naru stood up swiftly, dusting off her kimono, and blushed.

"Narusegawa . . ."

"Did you see?"

"No," I said quickly. "It was dark."

"So, your eyes were open?"

"I couldn't see anything!" I insisted. "Like, usually I glimpse your panties, but . . ."

Naru's lips quivered. She covered her face with her hands. "You saw!"

"No!"

She sniffled. "Kitsune told me I had to wear the uniform in a formal manner, so . . ."

So that meant no underwear. "Narusegawa . . ."

"So, so, so, y-y-you . . ." she blabbered.

"I didn't!"

She sobbed and punched me so hard I saw stars. It hurt, but maybe it was worth it, because an embarrassed Naru is definitely a cute Naru.

I went to the cafeteria, deep in thought. There, I saw Shinobu in tears. Her apron was about to fall off, and her kimono was wrinkled. Suu stood next to her, trying to cheer her up by making funny faces, but it wasn't working. Kitsune stood there, patting Shinobu's back.

"Shinobu?" I asked. "Why are you crying?"

She quickly wiped the tears off her cheeks, but new ones spilled down.

"What happened?" I pressed, worried.

"She was bullied," Suu replied.

"Bullied?"

"No," Shinobu said. "They got mad because I couldn't answer their questions."

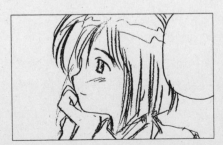

Shinobu had gone to serve Room 2—a group of four bachelors. When she went to retrieve the dishes and trays, they were fighting.

"They kept asking why Grandmother Hinata wasn't here. I told them she was traveling around the world. I also mentioned what you said, Keitaro, about her not wanting to ruin their image of the past by greeting them as she looks now."

I sighed.

"When I said that, they started taunting each other, saying, 'Oh, Hinata was in love with me,' and 'No, she wanted me, not you,' and so on."

When Shinobu had tried to stop their quarrel, they demanded she tell them which one she liked best. When she couldn't answer, they accused her of making fun of them, and caused a ruckus.

I understood Shinobu's predicament. Those four guys had a crush on Grandma Hinata; she must have been their goddess. Even now, they were still fighting over whom she liked the most.

Shinobu finally quieted down. "They asked me who was the most attractive. What could I say?"

"The richest guy is always the most handsome," Kitsune quipped.

Everyone laughed, except Shinobu.

I figured I'd better say something to those guys, so I headed toward the north building. On the way, I saw two men running away from Room 3. They rushed past me and made for the front entrance.

"Um, gentleman?" I asked.

From the hallway, I heard a voice thunder, "DIE!"

Motoko's energy wave (the blast of spiritual power that surrounds the blade of her sword) came right at me.

Why was she attacking customers?

WHOOM! WHOOSH! WHIZZZZ!

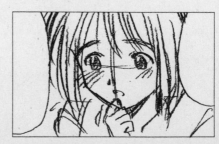

I didn't have time to react. The energy force struck me so hard that I slammed into the wall. Motoko dashed in front of me, her eyes burning a bright red.

"Um, what—?" But she ignored me, chasing after those two men.

I pulled myself together and rushed toward the front entrance, but the guys from Room 3 were long gone. The four guys from Room 2 and the elderly couple from Room 1 had packed up and were waiting to check out as well.

Naru and Shinobu, both near tears, bowed in apology, but the customers were adamant about leaving.

"Please stay?" Shinobu pleaded.

"Everything is under control now," Naru promised regretfully. She looked up at me and said, "Everyone says they're leaving early."

"But it's almost midnight!" I exclaimed. I approached one of the bachelors. "Sir, what happened? Is something the matter?"

"Definitely. I heard one of your staff swung a sword at a customer," he complained. "And the hot springs is full of weird fish!"

I was taken aback. I looked down at Suu, but she just scratched her head and laughed.

One lady complained, "The food trays flipped over. And also, one of your employees came on to my husband—right in front of me! Then she asked for fees for extra services!" She looked livid.

I glanced at Kitsune and sighed. I walked over to the front entrance, got down on my knees and said, "I'm really very sorry. I understand your frustrations. Please give us another chance. We will do our absolute best!"

It was embarrassing, but it seemed to convince them. They calmed down a little, at least.

"Keitaro," Shinobu said, smiling softly.

Naru placed her hand on my shoulder.

An old man with a white beard (the husband whom Kitsune had hit on) said, "It's our fault, too."

I tried to assure him that wasn't the case, but he wasn't paying any attention to me. Instead, he

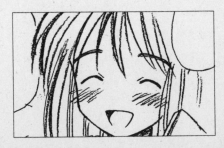

stared off at something far away. "We ended up comparing everything to the old Hinata Inn," he explained. "Hinata's strong leadership, the very pretty Miss Yoko, the well-trained staff." His eyes became misty. "There was something very special about the Hinata Inn."

The four bachelors nodded.

"This was a strange place. Every time we came here, something good would happen. To tell you the truth, I met my wife at this inn." He gestured to the elderly lady. "We were staying in separate rooms, but somehow, we were drawn to each other. Here, I was able to say and do things I'd normally be too nervous for. At Hinata Inn, I could open up to a total stranger."

The elderly woman glanced down, her face softening.

"But maybe that's just my imagination," the old man concluded. "People tend to embellish the past."

"No," one of the bachelors said. "When I came to the inn, my main reason was just to see Hinata once again. But to tell you the truth, whenever I stayed here, one of my fallen war buddies would come visit me in my

dreams. Or the person I shared rooms with had success with their business soon after . . ."

"Whenever our marriage was on the rocks, we'd come here to make up," the elderly lady said.

"Any business idea I came up with while here became an instant hit!" another said.

"I was able to reunite with someone I hadn't seen in a long, long time," offered yet another.

Someone else said, "No matter how bad things got, we could forget our troubles here."

Everyone nodded.

"Well, that's true for any vacation," Naru said softly. "Isn't it?"

"Yes," the old man conceded. "But we consider the Hinata Inn to be more than just an ordinary hot springs lodge. It was our mistake to expect this place to be as special as it was back in the day. I think it's best if we left."

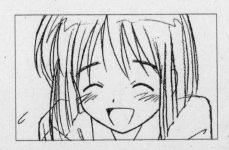

"No one is to blame," I said. "Thank you for everything."

The customers paid their bills and headed off for the train station. We couldn't keep them there any longer; we had no right to try and stop them.

What they'd said about the Hinata Inn stuck out in my mind.

To me, the Hinata House was my home. Just a very noisy girls' dorm. An everyday reality. Suu's inventions were fascinating, Motoko's sword skills were amazing, and Tama was just slightly odd. But we were a family, in a way. I'd never seen anything strange about this place.

I never sensed any special energy here. I couldn't understand what had attracted all those people to the Hinata Inn, and I doubted I'd figure it out any time soon.

Suddenly, I heard Kitsune scream, "Help, everyone! Come quickly!"

We dashed up the stairs to Motoko's room. Motoko was clad in pure white. Kitsune and Suu had pinned her down, but she was writhing on the floor.

At first glance, it was pretty obvious that Motoko was trying to commit *seppuku* (ritualized suicide). The

tatami mats were flipped upside down and Shisui was wrapped in white paper. I knew she practiced *bushido* (the samurai code of chivalry) but this was ridiculous.

"I have no excuse to offer you, Urashima," she said sadly. "I, Motoko Aoyama, have disgraced the Hinata Inn. I must pay for it with my life!"

"Don't even joke about it!" I told her.

"I'm not joking!" she insisted.

"Motoko feels responsible for the guests leaving," Shinobu said.

Well, she did instigate the mass panic, but honestly, after everything the old man had told me, I don't think it made that much of a difference.

"It's not your fault, Motoko." I sighed. "It's not good to swing your sword at people, but the customers left for their own reasons. It had nothing to do with how inexperienced we all were."

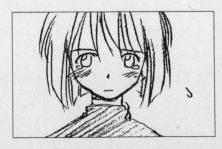

Motoko looked at me with teary eyes. It grabbed my heart. She looked so feminine and vulnerable right then. I was drawn to her . . .

"What the hell are you gazing at?" Naru asked.

"Nothing!" I said quickly.

Naru folded her arms. "Why did you chase after those guys anyway, Motoko?"

"Well," she began, "it was because they started talking about the treasure."

"Treasure? There's treasure?" Kitsune said, perking up. Her eyes sparkled.

"The Hinata House treasure, I mean," Motoko replied. "They said it had to be here."

"Didn't we just put that rumor to rest?" Shinobu asked.

Everyone looked at me. Or rather, tried to look at my back. The heat rash had long since disappeared.

"They knew the story about Urashima having a treasure map on his back," Motoko said. "I tried to laugh it off, explain that it was all a mistake, but they were really persistent. They swore they'd find the treasure."

"Did they have any proof?" Kitsune asked.

Motoko wrinkled her nose. "No. But, I mean, these customers had been coming here for twenty years. Back then, the old tower and the annex were off-limits. Still, they mentioned the treasure was supposed to be there."

At that time, I was barely a year old. Grandma Hinata warned me about the annex and tower when I was four, but she warned everybody about it long before then.

"They didn't state their source," Motoko said.

"That's not a lot to go on," Kitsune replied, losing interest.

"Why did you get so upset, Motoko?" Naru asked.

"It was such a ridiculous story. They were drunk, and kept bragging about how they were going to solve the riddle. I told them it was too dangerous to go there, especially since I sensed eerie energy. I tried to tell them there's nothing hidden in the annex, and that we'd already looked."

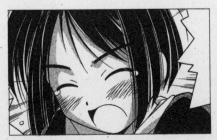

"The real treasure was Keitaro's crappy test scores!" Naru blurted out.

I was so embarrassed.

Naru shrugged, looking a little regretful. "So, then what?" she asked Motoko.

"They refused to believe me. They accused me of having found the treasure and said that I'd hidden it." She clenched her fists.

"We went back and forth about it, and then one of them reached out and grabbed my . . . my . . . my breast!"

Well. No wonder Motoko lost it! At this point, there was nothing we could do to bring the customers back, but I was starting to think that might not have been a bad thing.

What do we do now? I wondered. Everyone looked to me.

"What shall we do?" Naru asked me.

I shook my head.

Just then, the phone rang. I ran to the front entrance to answer it. It was Aunt Haruka. I had to wonder why she didn't just come on over from the teashop.

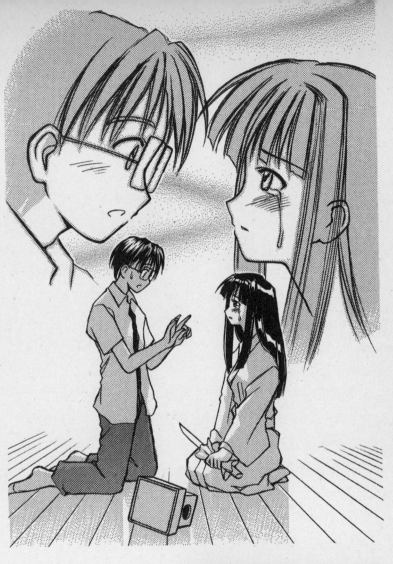

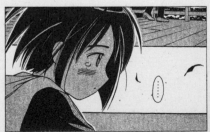

I figured she'd be angry about the guests leaving, so I said, "I'm sorry for letting you down. We really can't run an inn."

"What are you talking about?" she asked.

"Um . . . I thought you were calling because all the customers left."

"Oh, I noticed that. But never mind. Fresh start tomorrow! We still have other reservations."

I liked her tenacity, but I had to wonder what was up.

"So, I was wondering," she said. "Could you check out the front of my store?"

"You mean the teashop?"

"Yep. Since this afternoon, there's been a weird man lurking around. He sometimes stares into the shop window. I just want you to check it out for me."

"Are you sure it isn't an old acquaintance or something, Auntie?"

Aunt Haruka gritted her teeth and said, "Don't call me that. It's a much older guy. I've never seen him before. He looks a little familiar but—look, just in case, will you check it out?"

I decided to tease her a little bit. "Are you scared, Aunt Haruka?"

"Me? Of course not. But you've got a lot of pretty, young girls in the Hinata House. I worry about them."

She hung up the phone. I instantly felt guilty and decided I'd go take a look.

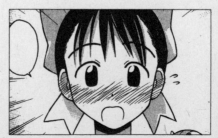

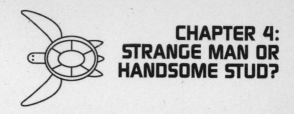

CHAPTER 4:
STRANGE MAN OR
HANDSOME STUD?

I wore my wooden sandals when I went outside. There were stone steps leading from the Hinata House to the teashop. I clacked my wooden shoes as loudly as I could. If there really was a weirdo out there, I didn't want to risk any chance encounters.

The teashop's shutters were closed. The whole building was wrapped in darkness. There wasn't much light coming from the Hinata House or the lamppost along the stone steps.

No one was there. I sighed in relief. I wasn't about to go searching through the vegetable garden behind the shop. It was dark and I was liable to break my neck. Now I could return, report that I'd seen no one, and just get some sleep.

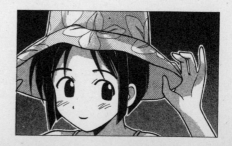

Just then, a shadowy figure appeared.

My scream died in my throat.

A man stood on the stone steps. He was skinny, maybe fifty years old. He had sunken shoulders and slightly bent knees. Despite the warm season, he wore a dirty coat and a plain tee shirt underneath. He looked at me with sad eyes. His face had deep wrinkles. I'm not kidding; he looked like a zombie.

His fingers and shoes were covered in dirt. Like he'd just crawled out of his grave.

"Hi," he said.

Okay. Zombies? Not big on the casual salutations. Weird.

"Where did you come from?" I asked.

He sighed, looking back and forth between the Hinata House and the teashop. "I didn't know where the entrance was, so I kept circling the area."

"Oh. Are you a customer? For the Hinata Inn?"

The man nodded.

I finally put two and two together. There was a gap in the vegetable garden that led to the stone steps. He was probably covered with dirt because

he'd accidentally stumbled into the garden and lost his way.

I had almost freaked out, thinking he was a ghost. But seriously, which is scarier—a ghost or a stalker?

I knocked on the teashop's door.

Aunt Haruka said, "Was he there?"

"He's a Hinata Inn customer," I replied.

The storm shutter opened an inch. Haruka looked suspiciously at the strange man. His eyes were fixed right on her.

"This is the teashop," I said. "Not the inn."

"Oh." He chuckled. "I thought it was the entrance to the inn!"

I nodded. He'd have to be practically blind to get the two confused, but I didn't feel like arguing. Aunt Haruka slammed the door shut without reply.

I led him to the inn's entrance and logged his name (Soujiro Natsuki) into the guest book. He'd made a

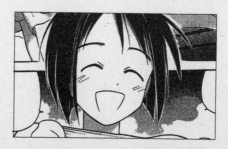

reservation, but arrived a day early. I called Naru to make sure Room 1 was clean, and then showed him to the north building.

"Are you mocking me?" Motoko demanded. She strode up to where I was sitting in the cafeteria, a tray of food poised precariously on her right hand.

"What's wrong?" I asked. "Mister Natsuki is in Room 1, waiting for his breakfast."

"I went to deliver it as you'd asked, but the customer was nowhere in sight!"

"Huh?" I scratched my head.

"You're taking advantage of my guilt about making the customers leave, aren't you?" Motoko said suspiciously. She added, "You're trying to fool me by making me run errands for imaginary guests, aren't you? I'll—"

Motoko somehow pulled out her replica sword with her left hand and held it over her head.

Fantastic. I can't even get breakfast before the beatings begin.

"What are you saying?" I swallowed. "Natsuki checked in late last night," I told her. "Narusegawa saw him too. Where's she? Ask her."

Shinobu answered, "She's cleaning the bath."

"Oh man. Come on, Motoko. Let's get to the bottom of this."

We went to Room 1. Just before we opened the door, I wondered if maybe I'd just imagined Natsuki. Maybe I'd dreamt up a false customer. These days, it was getting harder and harder to tell reality from my weird fantasies.

I hesitated, so Motoko opened the door instead.

Strong sunlight streamed in through the blinds. Natsuki was seated in the wicker chair next to the window. The air conditioner was on, but he was sweating something fierce. Had he been sunbathing?

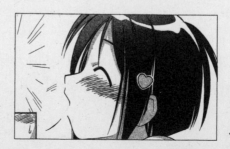

I smiled at Motoko. She relaxed a little and bowed before our guest. "I apologize for the delay. Here is your breakfast."

"Thank you. I was really hungry," Natsuki happily replied. He sat on the cushion at the breakfast table.

"Were you outside?" she asked, studying him closely.

"No. I've been in here the whole time." He slurped his miso soup loudly.

"But—" Motoko said.

I interrupted her, saying, "Sir, did you know we have *yukatas* in the closet? They're much cooler in the summer . . ." I stopped in mid-sentence.

Strangely enough, a yukata had been thrown over the futon—Natsuki had slept in it and then changed into his own clothes this morning. Well, it wasn't my place to question the odd habits of our guests. After all, he was the only customer we had right now, and I didn't want to run him off too.

We left. Motoko and I both stood in front of Room 1, staring at the door.

"See?" I said, breaking the silence. "Natsuki was right there."

"But he lied about going outside."

I shrugged. "Maybe he went to the bathroom or something. He doesn't need to explain himself to us."

Motoko shook her head. "There's something strange about his aura."

His aura? What, did he smell bad?

"Did you not sense it?" she asked me. "It felt the same as the old annex."

Natsuki's sudden appearance last night came instantly to my mind. He didn't just look tired—he seemed eerie and otherworldly when I met him. Maybe Motoko was right . . .

There was the sudden sound of rapid footsteps. Suu and Sara ran up to us, laughing. I braced for a full-body tackle, but instead they stopped in front of us and yelled, "The customers are here!"

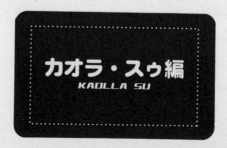

カオラ・スゥ編
KAOLLA SU

Today was the exact opposite of yesterday. Instead of a few guests, there was a mob crowding the Hinata Inn entrance. (Roughly thirty people, maybe more. Some of them couldn't fit inside the foyer and so they waited on the steps outside.)

"Wow! This is amazing," Kitsune said. "Come on!" Still clad only in her underwear, she tried to pull a handsome young man to the front of the line.

"What are you doing, Kitsune?" I cried. I turned to the customer. "I'm sorry, sir. Please wait your turn."

Naru and Shinobu split up and took the customers' names. Unfortunately, none of these people had a reservation.

Shinobu looked worried. One customer grinned down at her. "Gosh, I've never seen such a cutie before!" he said, grabbing Shinobu's hand.

She shrieked. Motoko cut between them and pushed the guy back outside. She turned around and glared at

all the customers, but they just locked eyes on her and started drooling.

"Ooooh!" they all said, pulling out their disposable cameras and snapping pictures of her.

"So, the rumor was true," one customer said.

"Yep! They're really hot!" another marveled.

"Do you think they perform special services?"

"They're promotion models, they ought to!"

"Heh heh, oh man!"

Something was seriously wrong with these guys. Suddenly, I saw my old classmates. They were in disguise, wearing knit caps and dark sunglasses, but they couldn't fool me.

"Shirai! Haitani!" I called. "I *told* you, there's no treasure!"

"We know," Shirai said. "But we're here for a different reason."

Haitani thrust a flyer at me. "Here, look at this."

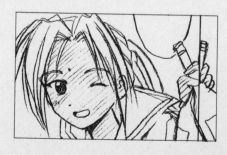

It said: *The Inn with Beautiful Girls—Four Days Only!* and there were hand-drawn caricatures of Naru and Motoko.

Who drew this crappy ad for the Hinata Inn?

If I was a clueless guy that had heard about a bunch of hot babes working for four days only at an inn with special services, I'd zip right on over here, too. *Did all these guys come here just for the girls?*

"Why couldn't you give us a heads-up on this, man?" Haitani asked. "We're big fans of Naru and Kitsune, you know—"

"And Haruka, too," Shirai added. (I think he had a thing for older women.) "Will they scrub our backs? They'll eat with us, right?"

"You guys!" I groaned. I had no clue what was going on. "Kitsune!" I called out.

She was posing in front of the crowd. When she heard me call her name, she sped away, quick as lightning.

"Somebody, catch her! Naru, get her!" I shouted.

"What about the customers?" Naru calmly asked.

"They don't have reservations, so, we need to make them move along."

The crowd didn't like that very much. I couldn't blame them. If I'd found a cute girl willing to provide special services, I'd jump at the chance, too . . .

I took a deep breath and addressed the group, "Excuse me, everyone! Please, you must leave!"

Nobody moved an inch. They kept trying to squeeze through the foyer.

I raised my voice and implored them, "Please understand, this isn't really an inn!"

"It's an inn, all right," one of the men said. He was gruff with huge muscles. "If not, how come you guys are dressed like that?" He pointed at Shinobu's apron and kimono.

"Please leave," I insisted.

The big guy took off my glasses and grabbed me by the hair. "Shut up, you little weasel! Let us stay!"

I was paralyzed with pain and fear.

Naru called out, "Keitaro!" She rushed forward and tried to yank me away from the man.

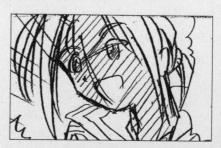

"Narusegawa," I murmured. "Ow ow ow ow, stop it, Naru!"

The guy clutched my hair, and she clutched my hips, and both of them tugged until I was ready to cry.

"Let go of Keitaro!" Naru ordered, placing her hand on the guy's arm.

He raised his left hand to punch her. I screamed, "Naru, run!"

BONK!

The guy that had me by the hair fell over on top of me. I was almost crushed under all that weight. I could just barely make out a guy in a suit. Two other handsome boys stood behind him, ready to back him up.

Apparently, Suit Guy had kicked Mister Muscles in the back.

Judging by their faces, they seemed to be in their early thirties. They had expensive suits and watches. Suit Guy looked foreign. He was really handsome. He dressed like a corporate businessman, but he didn't wear a tie, and his hair was a little long and wavy. To be honest, I had no clue what such a guy would do for an occupation.

"Don't lay your hands on the lady," Suit Guy told Mister Muscles. He reached out his hand and helped Naru up.

Naru blushed. I wondered why her eyes got all big and sparkly. She never shows that face to me. Never.

"Thank you very much," Naru said in a soft voice.

"No problem," Suit Guy said. He turned to the mob. "What's all this anyway? You guys are troubling the ladies. They've told you they can't lodge you. If you consider yourselves men, leave! This is a hot springs resort town. You can find rooms someplace else!"

The crowd readily obeyed.

I hated Suit Guy instantly.

He said just the right things at exactly the right time, in a calm and dignified manner. The crowd shuffled out and order was restored. I should have thanked him, but it was all I could do to find my glasses and keep from babbling idiotically.

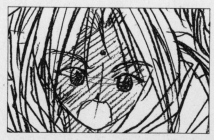

Kitsune, Shinobu, even Motoko stared in awe of Suit Guy. Even Suu said, "He's a stud, ain't he?"

Yeah. Regular stud muffin deluxe. Even I had to admit it.

I always knew that girls never considered me, but to see them respond to Suit Guy like he was God's gift to the world, well . . . It made me want to crawl into a hole and pull the hole in after me.

"Hey, Urashima," Haitani said. "We can stay, right?"

"We're friends, right?" Shirai asked.

I ignored them. *Losers*.

Suit Guy said to his companions, "Well, we should go too, gentlemen." They started to leave.

"Wait! You're our customers!" Kitsune said, rushing up to them.

Suit Guy smiled. "We heard there were beauties on the staff here, but I never expected anyone so lovely. Unfortunately, we didn't make reservations, so . . ."

"Oh, we can take care of that, can't we, Urashima?" Kitsune asked sweetly, her eyes pinning me to the floor.

In fact, everyone stared at me. Man, talk about pressure. "The other customers' reservations—"

"Most of them already left, remember?" Kitsune countered.

"The next customer will arrive soon," I said weakly.

"Natsuki only made a reservation for today," Shinobu offered politely. "The other reservations aren't until tomorrow!"

Thanks, Shinobu, I thought. *You're so honest.*

"But—" I was running out of counter-arguments. I looked to the other girls for help, but everyone seemed to really want these guys to stay.

"Let's put them up for the night, Keitaro," Suu said.

"We have plenty of food," Shinobu encouraged.

"And we owe them our gratitude," Motoko reminded.

Then Naru looked at me with pleading eyes and said, "Isn't it all right, Keitaro?"

I gave up.

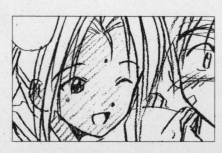

Suit Guy's name was actually Takeshi Kodaira. He told me he ran a small company in Hinata City. He was supposedly a young business owner. His companions were his employees.

Kitsune's eyes were glinting like a hunter watching a herd of game.

I didn't like these guys, but they were clean cut and polite, I had to admit. I'm not sure Kitsune would be able to seduce them so easily.

Kodaira complimented Motoko as she guided them to the cafeteria, and then chatted to Naru about her choice of tea. They teased Kitsune about her Osaka accent, and softly patted Shinobu's head as she served them.

Aware that they didn't have a reservation, after their light meal, they just stayed in their rooms and hung out. Suu finally urged them to come out, and then Kitsune and Motoko argued over who would give them the tour.

Watching the girls get so worked up made me uncomfortable. I kinda got distracted, thinking about it. I went around the inn, doing my chores, trying to figure out why these guys in suits bothered me so much. When I went to put the shampoos and soaps in the main bath area, I'd totally forgotten that it was the specified time for employee baths, and I just threw open the door.

"EEEEEEK!"

There were four silhouettes in the steam—Naru, Shinobu, Motoko, and Suu. The mist and the towels didn't completely shroud them from view, either. I could tell they were all in their birthday suits.

Naru and Motoko's eyes blazed. Shinobu started to cry. Suu looked like she was ready to jump all over me (in her usual manner of greeting me). I turned around immediately, but the image was burned forever into my brain. I'm a guy, okay? I can't help it.

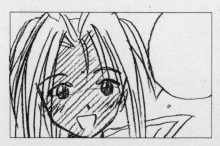

Suu ran around Motoko and Naru and then hurtled toward me. "Keitaro, are you gonna join us?"

She was a spunky kid, that's for sure. And she was developing nicely. But c'mon, I'm not *that* sick. I stammered and froze up as she pushed me toward the bath.

Shinobu had turned red from head to toe. She submerged herself almost completely underwater.

Motoko used her energy wave to stir the hot bath water up into a whirlpool. Suddenly the water convalesced and came at me in one big giant wave.

"You pervert!" Naru yelled.

"I will punish you!" Motoko swore.

Both girls punched me in the nose, and then the wave carried me back to the baths' entrance.

"Get out right now!" Naru yelled.

The door slid open. Kodaira stuck his head in. "Are we not allowed in yet?"

Couldn't they read the sign? I wondered.

I smiled. The girls would accuse these guys of being perverts too, and then I wouldn't have to take the brunt of their anger alone.

I waited for the infamous Naru Punch, but instead, Naru calmly said, "Oh, sorry. We'll be out soon."

I couldn't believe my ears. No Naru Punch? No screaming? No tears?

Kodaira played it cool, bowing. "Please forgive us. I'm very sorry."

Motoko quickly replied, "Well, it wasn't intentional."

"We were the ones taking too much time," Shinobu said.

"How about you join us?" Suu said, running toward them.

But they didn't freeze up like I had. They simply turned around and headed for the changing room, ignoring Suu completely.

I was confused. All healthy males would stop dead in their tracks if a naked girl ran toward them. And it was absolutely fitting that they get a Naru Punch or two.

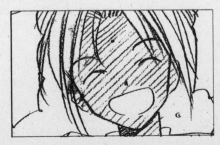

"Come on, Keitaro, get out already!" Motoko yelled.
"Idiot!" Naru screamed at me.

I wandered aimlessly around the hallways, my shoulders slumped. I stopped short when I saw Natsuki outside, sitting on the stone steps. His shoulders were even more slumped than mine. You know, he wasn't that bad of a guy. A little creepy, but . . .

Natsuki stared at the Hinata teashop. He was looking into the store windows. At first, I thought he was just relaxing in the sun, dozing off, but he didn't move so much as a millimeter the whole time.

Even though it was the end of the September, it was still really hot. You'd think he'd want to stay in an air-conditioned room, or at least lie back in the shade. But he just sat there in the sun, looking at the teashop, staring at Aunt Haruka.

Natsuki must have come to the Hinata Inn at some point in the past, since he was one of the guests that had made a reservation with Grandma Hinata. But he hadn't said

a word (thankfully) about how nostalgic everything was. In fact, he'd said very, very little.

"What are you doing?" someone suddenly asked me.

I twirled around, surprised. Kodaira stood behind me. He was alone. He must have taken a hot bath, because under his yukata, he was slightly sweating.

"Watching over our customer in Room 1," I explained.

"Ah, yes. I met him on the inner lawn."

"The inner lawn?" I repeated.

"There's an annex there, right?" Kodaira asked intently. "Mister Natsuki keeps staring at that teashop. Does he know something?"

" 'Know something?' " I tilted my head to the side, clueless.

"You should be careful of people like that." Kodaira patted my back and walked away.

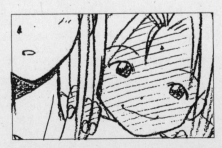

Well, he seemed like a nice guy. For a smooth-talking stud muffin, that is.

I looked outside the window, but Natsuki was gone.

I thought Natsuki seemed odd, and it wasn't just because Kodaira hinted at it. I went to go look for Natsuki, and Shinobu told me that she'd seen him head toward the main bath.

I poked my head into the changing room. Natsuki was there all by himself. I was curious, so I disrobed and joined him in the bath.

At first he didn't notice me. He just kept fiddling with the faucet and washing his fingers with lots of soap. He washed his arms, then went back to his fingers. Briefly, I wondered if he had OCD.

He must be a clean freak, I thought. He was so intense about it. His hands were almost black with dirt. I remembered that he was covered in dirt last night,

too, but I thought it was because he'd gotten lost in the garden.

Suddenly, Natsuki turned around. "Oh," he said, smiling. "You."

"Um . . . I'm staff, sir, but I didn't have a chance to take a bath earlier. Do you mind me being here? Do you want me to scrub your back?"

Natsuki waved his hand and politely declined.

We engaged in some small talk for a while, but then I blurted out, "You were looking at the teashop all day."

Natsuki looked surprised, but he nodded. "There's a young lady there."

"You mean Auntie Haruka?" I shivered. (Every time I say "Auntie" I immediately expect to get pummeled afterward.)

"She looks familiar."

"I heard she looks like my grandma. She'd probably get angry about that if I told her, though."

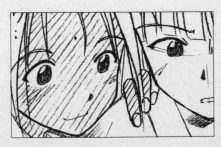

"Oh, yes," Natsuki said, nodding. "She does look like the inn mistress. But I think she looks even more like Yoko."

I blinked, suddenly remembering that Aunt Yoko was Haruka's mom. "Did you know Aunt Yoko?" I asked.

"A long time ago," he replied. "And only for a few months."

I'd only seen Aunt Yoko in photos, so I was curious about Natsuki's story. He talked about when Aunt Yoko was a student, forty-some-odd years ago. He said the climate was mild at the Hinata Inn, and sick people used to flock there to recover. As a child, I saw a number of guests come with different ailments, so that made sense.

"Back when I was a student," Natsuki said, "I failed the college entrance exams twice."

Wow. He's just like me, I thought.

"Of course, I didn't study much, but, I was also pretty sick," he continued. "My parents were worried about me, so they forced me to come here and relax."

According to Natsuki, the annex was used to house long-term visitors and sick patients. It was kinda like an

infirmary. Grandma Hinata left Aunt Yoko in charge of the annex and its guests.

"At first, I really hated being there," Natsuki said. "The annex looked like something out of a horror movie. Yoko was still a student, and she was too busy to manage everything. I wanted to run away. Not just from the annex, but from my third time taking that entrance exam."

That hit close to home.

"One day, I actually tried to escape. I ran to the train station with just the clothes on my back. My feet wouldn't take me any farther. I stood there, stuck on the platform. I couldn't think of anywhere to go. There was nothing for me at my house. So I ended up returning to the Hinata Inn. It was midnight by the time I got back."

He smiled. "A warm meal was waiting for me when I returned to my room. I was surprised. It was like Yoko was expecting me. She brought in a rice pot

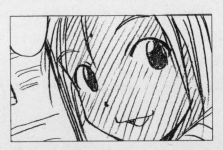

and quietly served me herself. I couldn't eat much, but I was happy."

Natsuki suddenly laughed. "When I finished, she asked if I was done, and when I said yes, she slapped me. Hard." He held his cheek and chuckled.

I could picture Aunt Yoko slapping him the same way I could see Haruka laying into me.

I waited for him to continue his story, but Natsuki just stepped out of the bath and headed for the changing room.

I followed him. "What happened to college?"

"After I stayed here, I got better, studied, and passed. Strange, isn't it?"

Once again, someone was calling the Hinata House strange. Maybe it was, but I'd never thought so.

"Aunt Yoko passed away," I said gently.

"Yes."

Natsuki's shoulders slumped again. Briefly, I wondered if he'd actually died ages ago, and really did crawl out of his grave every night, to haunt the Hinata House in search of Aunt Yoko.

But that was impossible. I couldn't see through him. He ate real food. And would a ghost bother to log his name in the guest book?

Even so, as I watched him go, I thought maybe there was something special about him, and this place.

"Oh, we'll service you!" Kitsune said, trying to hug Kodaira.

"Whoa, there!" Kodaira exclaimed. "No need to get so excited!" He didn't seem troubled, really, but he also didn't seem all that interested in Kitsune.

The man had to be a eunuch.

Motoko happily poured drinks for Kodaira and his employees. (I wondered if hell had frozen over.)

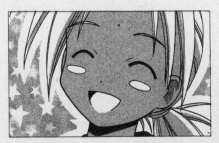

Kodaira smiled. "Wow, a Japanese beauty pouring me a drink. I've died and gone to heaven! I hope I don't get drunk, off the sake, or your loveliness."

Motoko blushed and murmured thanks.

Shinobu brought in a set of dishes. She seemed extra perky. Every time someone said "delicious" or, "you'll make a great cook," or, "I wish I had a girl like you," she'd smile shyly. Sometimes she looked over at me, but she never said a word.

Suu and Sara put on strange (and far too revealing, if you asked me) costumes and sang and danced for the guests.

And Naru . . . She was letting one of Kodaira's employees read her palm!

"Oh really?" she cooed.

"Yeah, it's true. That's the life line, and this is the love line."

Even I could tell this whole fortune-telling thing was just a ploy, an excuse to touch Naru. Why was she letting him do that?

He told her, "You will meet a special person soon."

I just about gagged. Palm reading was so bogus.

But no one seemed to care. It was a regular old party at the Hinata Inn, let me tell you. It was like Christmas, a picnic, and Golden Week all rolled into one. The alcohol flowed. The food was delicious. The girls wore pretty kimonos. Oh, what a sight. Just like I'd always dreamed it would be.

Except no one was paying the slightest attention to me.

See, in my fantasy, the Hinata House was an inn, and all the girls were fighting to hook up with me. I was a brilliant Todai student, living the sweet life. The girls would say things like, "I always wanted a Todai boyfriend," or, "Please be my mentor and teach me everything you know," or, "Do whatever you'd like with me!"

Instead, I just sat there, watching the girls fawn all over Suit Guy and his lackeys. Every once in a while, I'd mutter things like, "Kitsune, don't get so close to them,"

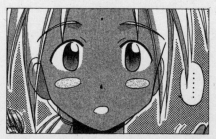

or, "Suu, don't spread your legs like that!" I sounded like an evil mother-in-law or something. Not that it mattered, since no one listened to me.

I couldn't take it anymore. I stood up, grabbed Naru's arm, and led her out of the room. "Hey!"

"What? We're working." Her smile faded and she glared at me.

"You call that work?" I said shrilly.

"What do you mean? It's not as if we're giving them a lap dance or anything. And Kodaira isn't a pervert, unlike some people I might mention."

"What?" That had hurt.

Naru huffed. "We finally have well-mannered customers. We need to give them our best service. And Kodaira's compliments . . . well, they make me happy. What's wrong with that?"

"You know what will happen if you let him keep going," I said.

Naru blushed. "They won't do a thing. It's harmless flirting. Let's go back already."

"No!" I gripped her arm harder. "Why? You're eager to get back in there, aren't ya?"

Naru tilted her head. "Keitaro. *You're* the one that asked us to help you run the inn. Now you want us to just quit?"

"W-well . . ." I didn't know what to say. It's not like I could order her not to touch those guys. Instead, I said, "Someone has to take care of Natsuki in Room 1."

Naru narrowed her eyes.

Just then, Kodaira poked his head out of the room and chuckled. "Shouldn't you just let that old guy alone?" He gently snaked his arm around Naru's waist and led her back inside.

I could only follow. "What do you mean leave him alone? He's a valuable customer."

"He's suspicious," Kodaira fired over his shoulder.

We sat down, and Kodaira's employees piped in, "His hands were dirty this afternoon."

"He kept staring at the teashop like he was casing the joint."

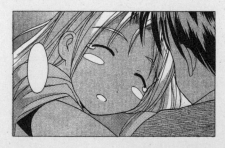

Kodaira sighed. "I don't know. But maybe . . .
Do you girls know about the rumor concerning the
Hinata Inn?"

"You mean the treasure?" Motoko asked, irritated.

"Yes, that," Kodaira said. "That rumor spread all the
way out to our store, and we're down by the train station.
There are tons of people who believe it."

Shinobu looked depressed. I guess she didn't want
to believe that a former inn customer would only come
here to steal treasure.

"That rumor is completely false," Motoko said flatly.

Kodaira peered at her. "Really? Too bad. But you
know, the people that believe it aren't the kind of people
that will listen to reason. Besides, you guys haven't
checked the annex from top to bottom, have you?"

"Well, no, but . . ." Naru hesitated.

He nodded. "Anyway. You should be more careful
around that creep. He's posing as an old customer, but
he acts awfully strange."

"I don't think he's a weirdo," I jumped in. "When
I talked to him in the baths, Natsuki didn't seem like a
calculating person."

"Oh?" Kodaira swept me with his eyes. "Well, why do you think he was digging around and checking out the buildings?"

Because he's a ghost, I thought. But I couldn't just blurt that out. So, instead, I drank a bottle of sake until it was dry. Pretty soon, I got bored with the party, so I went out into the hallway.

My vision narrowed. I felt like I'd already got a hangover. I don't usually get drunk, but I was depressed.

Why did it have to turn out like this? I couldn't refuse Grandma Hinata's request to reopen the inn. And it *was* my idea to involve the girls. But this just sucked.

The first batch of customers had run away. The second group monopolized the girls. And worst of all, the girls seemed to enjoy it!

I wasn't as talented as Grandma; I couldn't make this inn famous. I couldn't even get it to run smoothly.

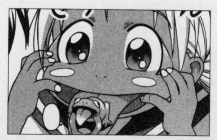

Whatever magic used to be on these grounds, it was gone now.

Things always turned out like this. I couldn't stand it anymore. I stormed off to Room 1.

Was Natsuki really here to dig up treasure? Did he totally make up all that stuff he'd told me about in the baths? I needed to find out.

Angry and drunk, I barged my way into Natsuki's room, but he wasn't there.

A used yukata once again lay on top of the futon. I guess he couldn't dig wearing the robes. He must have been digging this morning too. That's why he was wearing a ratty old tee shirt.

WHUMP!

I dropped to my knees. I couldn't move my legs. I tried to push myself up, but it was no use. Something was terribly wrong. I'd never been this drunk before. I tried to call for help, but my tongue wouldn't work.

My vision got dark. All I could make out was the woven straw of the tatami mat. Then, everything went totally black . . .

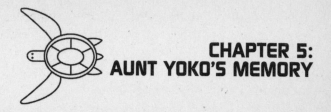

CHAPTER 5:
AUNT YOKO'S MEMORY

"**K**eitaro, I'm sorry!" Naru said as she embraced me. Her kimono melted away, but for some odd reason, the apron stayed on. (She was so much sexier with just a few articles of clothing on.) When we hugged, I could feel her soft skin.

We kissed passionately, but I broke away, playing hard to get.

"Why are you apologizing, Narusegawa?" I whispered.

She looked embarrassed. "Because, even though I have a wonderful man like you, I wanted Kodaira's attention!"

"I know," I said, a little coldly.

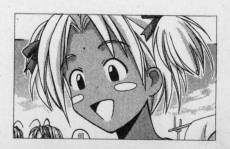

"Keitaro," she pleaded.

I pressed my lips to hers, kissing her deeply, my hands tangling into her hair.

This was only my third kiss, if you counted Mutsumi in Okinawa, and my accidental kiss with Naru on the beach. Still, I was an expert at it.

Naru slipped her tongue into my mouth. It was thick and hard, pushing deeper and deeper into my mouth. I tried to spit it out, but Naru had me in a headlock and wouldn't let up. I couldn't breathe! I clamped my teeth together . . .

"Myu!"

My eyes snapped open. Tama was glaring at me. There were small scars on his neck.

I'd passed out in Room 1. My mouth tasted like salt and smelled like turtle.

"Ugh. Tama, I'm sorry I bit you, but man, you shouldn't do that!"

Tama held up a little sign that said, "It hurt!" Then he ran out into the hallway (as fast as a turtle could run).

I didn't feel drunk anymore. I was able to move about. I got up and went into the hallway.

Everything was dark and quiet. I wondered how long it had been since I'd fallen asleep.

Tama scurried past Room 3 and headed for the stairs. I stopped and took a quick look inside. Leftover food and drinks were scattered about, but aside from Kitsune, who lay there, snoring loudly, everyone else was gone.

On closer inspection, she didn't look quite right. I shook her gently. "Kitsune? Anything wrong? Where did everyone go?"

She murmured, "Go ahead, Keitaro," and spread her legs wide open. The kimono slid away and I could see her milky white thighs.

I remembered that she wore her kimono in the formal fashion, and I gasped.

Suddenly, Tama cried, "Myu!"

I fixed Kitsune's kimono and closed her legs, wondering where the heck Naru and the others had gone.

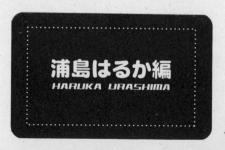

浦島はるか編
HARUKA URASHIMA

Tama trudged out of the north building and headed straight for the pond. He floated over toward the annex.

For a second, I worried that the party had gotten really wild, and that everyone paired up and headed to separate rooms. I checked each room just to be sure, but the girls weren't there either. Plus, if anyone was going to hook up with the guests, it would have been Kitsune.

Then I thought of something dreadful. *What if Kodaira was right, and Natsuki really was looking for treasure? What if he'd somehow drugged our drinks, made us pass out, and kidnapped the girls? What if he left Kitsune and locked the rest of them up somewhere?*

I prayed for Naru and everyone else's safety.

Tama got out of the pond and made for the entrance to the annex. He kept going, "Myu myu!" so I decided to follow him.

A thin ray of light shone in the foyer. I heard mumbling and rustling. Someone was definitely in there.

Well, the front door wasn't the only way in.

A few minutes later, I'd climbed atop the roof. (Tama rode on my shoulder.) Thick clouds concealed the moon. It was really dark. I kinda felt like a ninja or something. It was a long way down. I could just barely make out the ripples on the pond below.

At this point, I was covered in scratches and bruises, but it didn't matter. I flipped back the blue tarp that covered the hole the Mecha Tama had made, swung my legs over the side, and carefully jumped down the hole. Unfortunately, there were several feet between the ceiling and the floor, and I crashed down pretty loudly.

"Ow ow ow!" I bit my hand and tried to keep my voice down.

Suddenly, in the darkness, I could make out a scary face—a scrawny, wrinkled, leathery face. Dark eyes stared at me.

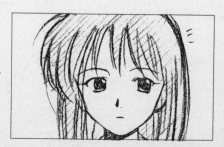

I almost fainted.

Then I realized it was Natsuki.

I backed away, but there was nowhere to run or hide. I was unarmed, and a little banged up, and way scared. So I just grabbed Tama and pointed him at Natsuki like he was a gun. Hey, it was dark. Maybe he couldn't see that it was a turtle.

"Don't move!" I commanded.

"Shh!" Natsuki hissed. "Quiet."

I inched forward and took a good look at Natsuki. He was sitting on the floor, completely still. His hands were tied behind his back with kimono belts. I instantly forgot my fear.

"Are you all right?" I asked, going to him.

"For now," he replied, smiling without mirth. Odd noises came from downstairs. Natsuki nodded. "They're down below."

"Who?"

"I don't know. They were talking about treasure or something."

I untied Natsuki and helped him stand up. We moved to the hallway and peered down the staircase.

Several flashlight beams cut through the darkness, casting human shadows on the wall.

I held my breath and leaned farther over. I recognized one of the faces—it was one of Kodaira's employees!

"What did they say about treasure?" I whispered to Natsuki.

"When I was in the hallway, they jumped me. It happened so fast. They punched me and then tied me up. Then they said, 'We'll find the treasure all by ourselves!' or something." He looked at me. "Do you know what they were talking about?"

"It's just a silly rumor," I told him. "It doesn't exist. There is no treasure!"

I was now convinced that Natsuki didn't come to Hinata Inn to find the treasure. But I still had no clue why he'd come to the annex.

As if reading my mind, Natsuki said, "I was looking for something else here."

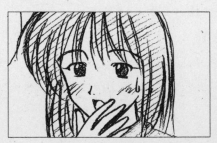

"What? Did you leave something behind on your last visit?" I asked.

"Perhaps I did forget something." He sighed. "I told you about how Yoko helped me get back on my feet, right? Once I got well and entered college, I passed the federal employee exam and went to work for the government. Then one day, I received a letter from the inn mistress."

"Grandma?"

"It was a very short letter to inform me of Yoko's death." He looked so sad.

I knew Aunt Yoko married in her late twenties and gave birth to Haruka, but soon afterward, she fell ill. She didn't live much longer after that. Her husband took Haruka and moved away from the hot springs town. After college, Haruka came back on her own. That's all I knew, really.

"I didn't even go to the funeral," Natsuki said, agonized. "It wasn't because I was overwhelmed with grief or sorrow or anything like that. I was simply too busy."

I sighed deeply.

"My job kept me really busy," he said, hanging his head. "Everything I did got me higher up the corporate ladder. I wanted to expand my network, branch out, become independent, and start my own business. By the time I'd received the inn mistress' letter, I'd completely forgotten about Yoko and all her kindnesses to me. What a jerk I was."

I couldn't say anything. I was a starving student who'd never been out in the real world—it wasn't my place to judge another person.

"I started thinking that I'd achieved everything all by myself," Natsuki whispered. "I took other people for granted. People were nice to me because I worked for the government office. My wife tried very hard to manage the house, because I was almost never home. I just figured it was her duty as my wife. I never thought about what it felt like for her. I was an ungrateful ass. To Yoko. To everyone."

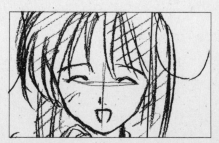

He smiled bitterly. "Do you really think success would last long, with that kind of attitude?"

Natsuki adjusted his collar. "When I set up my own business, it dried up within two years. In order to remove my wife's name from the debt, I divorced her. Perhaps that was the only favor I ever did her, really. I'm alone. All I have left of my fortune is this old coat."

I looked away.

"Then I remembered," he continued. "I remembered who got me on track in the first place. Who helped me go to college. It was at this inn—it was a young girl named Yoko. This place has a strange power. Whenever I come here, I reflect on my life, and I see miracles."

"Getting into college wasn't a miracle, Mister Natsuki," I said. "You worked hard for that."

He shook his head and looked at me. "To tell you the truth, boy, when I heard that I could come back to this old inn, I thought I might once again have a chance to change my luck. I hoped my failed business and my broken marriage would heal."

He trailed off, looking far away. "But nothing's happened." He sighed. "I thought, if I could just take

something, a memento . . . so I dug through the rubble.
But there was nothing. I started gazing at Haruka,
who looks so much like her mother. But Haruka
isn't Yoko. And this isn't the past. I've been in denial,
wasting time."

Suddenly it all made sense. "I'm sorry," I said.

He looked at me quizzically. "Why? *I'm* the one that
caused *you* trouble."

"Not really. This isn't the Hinata Inn anymore," I
said. "We all tried to do our best, but we're just students.
Whatever strange things may have happened here, it's
just a regular dorm now. There's no magic."

"Are you so sure?" Natsuki asked me. "When I
lived in the annex, I never sensed any strange powers.
But when I grew up a bit, I realized . . . The day I didn't
take that train . . . the relief I'd felt when I returned to
the Hinata Inn . . . the meal . . . Yoko slapping me . . .
I didn't think anything strange about that then. Now I

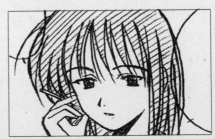

realize—those things were special. They changed my life. They meant someone cared for me."

I wasn't exactly convinced that the Hinata House had strange powers. I was a dorm manager, not a magician. But now was not the time for such esoteric thoughts. I had to make sure the girls were safe and get Kodaira and his goons out of here!

"Natsuki, where are the girls?" I asked.

He frowned. "I thought they were back at the inn . . . Well, now that you mention it, after I was tied up, I heard those guys say something about sleeping pills."

My heart raced. *So that's why I passed out. And why Kitsune wouldn't wake up. They must have put drugs in the drinks.*

But did Kodaira take the girls to another room, or did he tie them up somewhere like he'd done to Natsuki?

If they didn't find the treasure, would they try to get ransom for the girls, or sell them off as mail order brides to a foreign country?

NO WAY!

"I won't let that happen!" I bellowed.

"Wait! We have to call the police!" Natsuki said. He tried to hold me back, but I wrenched away from him.

I bolted for the stairs. "Naru!"

CRACK! RUMBLE!

I tumbled down the stairs and sprawled out onto the dirty floor. I hit my head hard and blacked out.

I woke, bleary-eyed and disoriented.

Kodaira loomed over me. "I guess the drugs were too weak."

I could see his men. They had picks and shovels. Suddenly I understood why they bullied the other customers away, and raised suspicions about Natsuki—they wanted to draw attention away from themselves so that they could check out the annex.

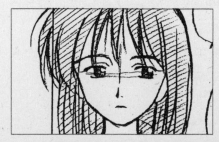

"Where's Narusegawa and the other girls?!" I demanded, struggling to my feet.

Kodaira kicked me back down. "They're dreaming pretty dreams, boy."

"Where did you put them?"

"Where's the treasure?" he countered.

I sighed. "I told you. There is none."

WHACK!

He slapped me upside my head with his shovel. Pain blossomed behind my eyes.

"If there is no treasure," Kodaira said, "then what's up with the annex and tower? Both are well built. How come you never fixed it up and used it again?"

Because we didn't have the money to fix it, dumb ass, I wanted to say. Instead, I told him, "Grandma Hinata must have her reasons."

Kodaira smiled grimly. "Nice try. Look, everyone knows that old people don't trust banks. If they have anything valuable, they hide it. There's no other reason for keeping the annex and the tower up—the taxes on the buildings alone must cost a fortune."

I was puzzled about that.

Suddenly, Natsuki stood at the top of the staircase and said, "There is no treasure!"

I looked up at him. He didn't look frail or lost anymore. He came down the stairs, glaring at Kodaira. "What do you know about human hearts, Mister Kodaira? The inn mistress probably kept these buildings because she had fond memories of them."

Kodaira snorted. "People will do a lot of things for money, old man. They don't waste it on silly memories."

"Just because you think so," Natsuki said caustically, "doesn't mean everyone else acts like that."

"Shut up!" Kodaira's eyes smoldered.

Natsuki continued down the stairs. "Why can't you leave things as they are? You shouldn't dig up the past."

"I told you to shut up!" Kodaira hissed. "I've had my eye on this inn for years. My family ran the real estate agency near the train station. We asked the inn mistress several times

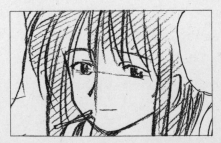

to sell us this land, but Granny never agreed. Dad always used to joke that she'd buried some treasure up here."

Kodaira's eyes narrowed. He gripped the shovel so hard his knuckles turned white. "Dad died. There was a recession. Our agency failed. I worked night and day, but nothing helped. All I could think about was the Hinata House treasure, how it could save our business."

Natsuki paled.

In a way, both of them came to the Hinata Inn to try and reverse their fortunes. This place seemed to attract people who were down on their luck.

"There has to be treasure here!" Kodaira insisted. "If there isn't, then I'm just a fool! I mean, I asked your staff, and everyone in town—they've all heard of the rumor. So . . . So, don't get in my way!"

"I understand how you feel," Natsuki murmured. "But there's nothing here anymore."

"Shut up!"

One of Kodaira's employees raised his pick and made to swing at Natsuki. I grabbed his legs, all the while dodging the other employee's shovel. I thought they really were going to kill me.

Suddenly, sparks sprayed from the ceiling. There was an explosion. All the flashlights cracked and sputtered out. The room went completely black. There was the faint smell of burnt plastic.

Kodaira's employees dropped their tools and tripped over each other, trying to run away.

"Turn on some lights!" Kodaira yelled.

Just then, a voice came out of nowhere: "LEAVE!"

It sounded like a woman's voice, but it was so strange.

Kodaira's employees flipped out, terrified. (For the record, if I hadn't recognized the voice, I probably would have wet my pants, too.)

"Where's it coming from?" Kodaira demanded, turning around several times.

"LEAVE!" the voice bellowed again, bouncing off every wall in the annex.

FLAP FLAP FLAP FLAP!

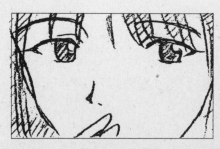

I heard something that sounded like the beating of a bird's wings. Then a portion of the wall cracked open. It was like something out of the movies. Suddenly dozens of bats flew out from the crack. They chased Kodaira's employees around.

"Aaaah!" Kodaira screamed. "Are they vampire bats? Get rid of them!"

I almost felt sorry for him. By now, I'd had enough experience with Suu's crazy inventions to know when I was looking at one of them. (Or dozens, in this case.) She'd made a bunch of Tama-sized flying robots. In the dark, they looked like scary bat monsters, but I could easily tell the difference.

(On the floor, the real Tama was bouncing up and down, trying to fly with the robots. Occasionally, he'd called out, "Myu!" as if to say hello.)

The front door slammed open. The voice thundered, "LEAVE!!!"

A woman clad all in white, with long dark hair draped over her face, suddenly appeared from out of the darkness. Blood trickled out of her mouth. In her hands, she held a long, gleaming sword.

That was scary enough all by itself. But it looked like she had several arms!

"It's a monster!" Kodaira's employees whimpered.

The woman slashed out at them, and *SNIP!* Their belts snapped off, their pants split, and the shreds fell to the ground. Speechless, the employees grabbed up their destroyed clothing and ran out of the building in their underwear.

I threw my head back and laughed. "Good job, Motoko!"

She glared at me. I heard several voices whisper and grumble.

Kodaira, who had overheard, stalked up to Motoko and wrenched back the sheet she'd been wearing, revealing Naru and Shinobu. Shinobu had a frying pan (I guess that was her idea of a weapon) and she pointed it at Kodaira.

He just smirked, pulled out a knife, grabbed hold of Naru, and held the blade under her throat.

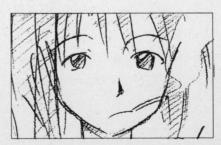

"That's a dirty trick!" Motoko yelled.

Shinobu started tearing up.

"You had us fooled, little girls," Kodaira said, panting.

"Aw, we almost had them," Suu said, coming out from behind the staircase. She held a remote control device and wore night-vision goggles.

Natsuki nodded and said, "Oh, yeah. I'd forgotten about the storage room under the stairs."

I sighed.

Kodaira looked livid. "So, what? You all acted drunk and beat us to the annex, huh? Tried to scare us away?" He chuckled. "When did you figure it out?" He tapped the flat of his blade on Naru's throat.

"In the morning," Naru said. "When we took you to your rooms. The first thing you asked about was the annex and the old tower. You weren't here because of those flyers."

"We took turns watching you," Motoko added. "You mentioned the rumor about the treasure and tried to make us suspect Natsuki."

"We knew from the start, you creep!" Shinobu shouted.

Wow. I guess the only clueless person in the room is me. "You guys should have told me, too!"

"How could we?" Naru said coldly. "You're a blabbermouth. You would have blown our cover. Besides . . ." She stopped, blushing a dark red.

"What?"

"Keitaro," she whispered. "How could you think we'd all fall for such jerks?"

I looked down ashamed. I'd underestimated everyone.

"The only person who was really into these guys was Kitsune, so we let her drink all the sake, and then acted the same way she did," Naru explained.

Oh, that was their way of lowering Kodaira's guard.

"I really hate how dense you are, Keitaro!" Naru yelled.

I couldn't think of any response.

"You can have this heartwarming chat later," Kodaira said. "First, tell me where the treasure is!"

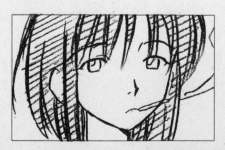

"There is no treasure, you dolt!" Motoko said, furious. "Get your hands off Naru!"

She pointed her sword at him, but Kodaira just used Naru as a human shield.

Now, Motoko had a special skill known as the *zanma ken,* which could pass through a person and obliterate whatever was behind them. But if Motoko tried it, she risked accidentally hurting Naru.

We couldn't do a thing.

"No more denying the truth!" Kodaira roared.

"You can't coerce us into making something up!" Motoko said indignantly.

Kodaira wouldn't listen. He turned to Natsuki and said, "Hey, Grandpa, what do you think? You came here for treasure. You probably already know where to look."

Natsuki didn't answer. He was shaking. Slowly, he pointed behind Kodaira.

I couldn't believe it. Was there actually a treasure, and Natsuki was going to hand it over to Kodaira?

We all looked over to where he pointed. What we saw was utterly unbelievable.

The rubble in the hallway was totally gone. The wallpaper was no longer peeling off; the chandelier was brightly lit, back up on the ceiling. The annex looked brand new.

"What's going on?" Naru asked, trembling. Shinobu gasped and Suu gulped.

Motoko took a step back. "This is exactly what I saw yesterday."

I'd seen it before, too. Back when I was four years old and I'd entered the annex without permission. It looked the same in every way.

"What kind of trickery is this?" Kodaira asked, stepping forward.

At the end of the hallway, a door opened. Until this moment, it had been entirely buried in rubble. It was the same door I had peeked in as a child . . .

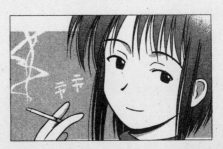

"No," Motoko whispered, shaking.

Kodaira ignored her and pushed Naru toward the door. They stepped inside . . .

I snapped out of my daze and dashed forward, desperate to get to Naru. But Natsuki beat me to it.

The door blasted open and Kodaira screamed. He stumbled back out of the room, horrified. He fled down the hall and out the front door. I kinda wanted to do the same thing, but Naru was too important to me to just leave behind.

"Narusegawa!" I yelled.

I entered the room, and the annex immediately returned to its original state. The lights went out. The walls were dirty. Piles of rubble cluttered the hallway.

Naru stood there, looking blankly at me.

"Narusegawa, are you all right?" I asked. "Naru?"

She started crying. "No, I'm fine. I'm a little sad . . . but also happy."

I wanted to comfort her, but I couldn't work up the nerve.

"What happened?" Natsuki asked.

"I don't know." She shook her head. "There was a woman in here. I was scared so I closed my eyes. Then I heard Kodaira scream. He left . . ."

"Well, that doesn't explain a thing," Suu complained. "Was the woman an evil spirit? Did you sense anything, Motoko?"

But Motoko didn't speak.

"It wasn't an *evil* spirit," Naru insisted.

Natsuki nodded, looking satisfied. Shinobu smiled.

Suddenly there was a warm, white light coming from the foyer. Everyone turned to look. A young woman that looked a lot like Aunt Haruka stood there. She smiled at Natsuki.

He tried to approach her, but she held up her hands.

I suddenly remembered something. The day I'd entered the annex and Grandma had scolded me, I'd called out for Auntie Haruka. I'd seen this woman at that

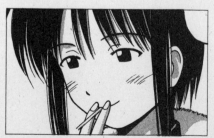

time. She'd raised her hands to me, motioning me to stop back then, too. Like she was trying to protect me.

Natsuki stood stock-still. The woman lowered her hands. Her body scattered like rain droplets and she disappeared.

"Yoko," Natsuki said, like he had to squeeze the word out.

The entrance door opened. Aunt Haruka walked in, wearing jeans, a tee shirt, and an apron from the teashop. "What the heck are you all doing here at this hour of the night? Your customers got caught streaking in public and were arrested by the police!"

We all let out a big, relieved sigh.

The next morning, Aunt Haruka wrung her hands. "Are you sure it's all right?" she asked.

"He's not really an oddball," I said.

"Oh yeah? Only an oddball would want to take a picture of an old woman like me."

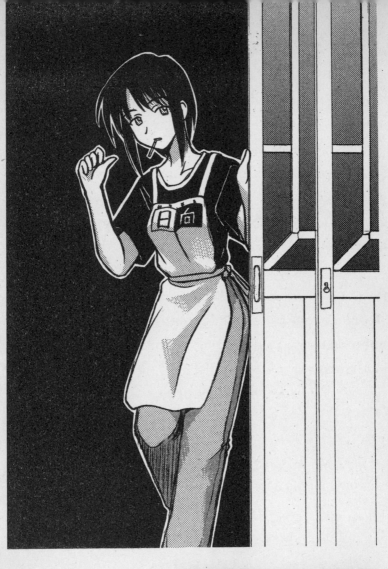
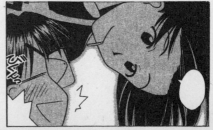

I smirked. Aunt Haruka was far from looking old, but even so, she didn't like having pictures taken of her. I wasn't sure why, but this time, I wouldn't back down.

"You look like Aunt Yoko. That's how come he kept staring at you. So come on. For old times' sake? Think of it as customer service," I said.

I dragged Aunt Haruka to the front entrance of the Hinata House. Natsuki was getting ready to leave. Naru came up to us and handed me a disposable camera.

I motioned for Aunt Haruka to stand next to Natsuki. "Closer. Closer," I said.

"It's not like we're a couple, Keitaro," she grumbled.

"Just for the picture. Please?"

Natsuki blushed. "It's all right, Urashima."

I wanted to give Natsuki the picture of them together as a gift. I suppose Aunt Haruka could never replace Aunt Yoko, but it was the least I could do.

Natsuki had decided to return home, rebuild his business, and try to get back together with his family.

I was certain this picture would help remind him of his goals.

"Come on, Aunt Haruka. Closer together now. And put out your cigarette." I stepped back, trying to get the best shot.

"Don't you think it's strange, Urashima?" Natsuki said, smiling. "Both Kodaira and I were saved by this place."

Natsuki had definitely felt renewed, but Kodaira? I'm not sure he was saved, and I said as much.

"Well, he didn't find treasure. But maybe what happened last night changed him," Natsuki wondered. "And since you didn't press charges against him, at the very least, his luck is improving."

I nodded and looked into the lens. The Hinata House fit in the viewfinder. Several faces were looking out of the windows—Kitsune, Shinobu, Sara, Suu, and Motoko.

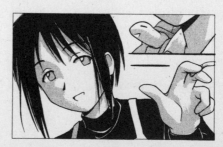

"I'll just back up a little more and get all you guys in," I said.

"Be careful," Naru warned.

"Keitaro!" Kitsune yelled. "Make sure I'm in the shot!"

Everyone laughed.

I smiled. I lived in a strange, but wonderful building, with some strange, but wonderful girls. I'm a loser and a failure and a klutz, and probably no power on Earth or from beyond the grave could change that. But this was my home, and everyone accepted me here, just as I was.

"Back up a little more!" Suu said.

I did.

"Oh dear!" Shinobu said.

"Keitaro!" Naru called.

I tumbled down the steps to the garden and landed face-first in the dirt.

Naru ran out of the building and down to the garden. I tried to get up, but wobbled so much that I almost fell over.

"Keitaro," Naru said, grabbing onto me and keeping me balanced.

"Thanks, Naru," I said, reaching out to steady myself.

Unfortunately (or perhaps fortunately?) my hand landed on Naru's left breast. I could feel her heartbeat in my palm. The faint vibrations sped up.

Her eyes narrowed. "Grow up already!"

KABOOM!

Her uppercut rocketed me into the sky. I could just barely make out her face as I soared. She was laughing. Maybe she was chuckling at how pathetic I am.

But, to see such a cute girl smile so brilliantly, well . . . even if I didn't get girls, I did get one thing—the Hinata House had some magic after all.

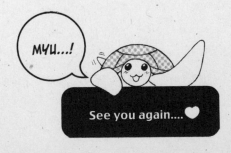

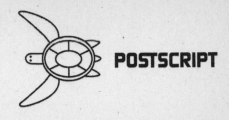

POSTSCRIPT

Good day! I'm Ken Akamatsu, creator of *Love Hina*.

Did you enjoy the first novel?

The author, Kurou Hazuki, is the scriptwriter for the *Love Hina* anime. He's a key member of the "Ani Hina" staff, and has probably read the *Love Hina* manga a million times, so I trust him a lot.

By the time this novel comes out, the manga will have taken a little break. I drew the novel illustrations before I went on vacation. I wanted a different look for the pressed art, so I didn't use any pens (not because I'm lazy), but instead used compressed pencil lines. I called my assistant to help me with zip tones, so it was kind of new and fresh. Doing illustration jobs can be fun.

Regarding Haruka's mother, Yoko, please take her character and situation as the official story, even for the *Love Hina* manga. However, the annex layout in the novel is quite different from the one in the manga. For future

things like that, I may need to invite Hazuki on a trip to a hot springs inn and we can meld our thoughts and visions! Of course, we'd expense it as a business trip!

Anyway, the first novel is complete. The anime and manga are finished.

Thank you for your support of *Love Hina!*

Love Hina PREVIEW

When a crazy robot that looks exactly like Keitaro appears out of the blue at the Hinata House, the tenants of the all-girls dorm band together to fend off the out-of-control "Mecha-Keitaro."

Meanwhile, Motoko struggles to show off her special skills in an effort to impress her sister, Tsuruko. But a secret spell ends in disaster as Motoko accidentally switches bodies . . . with Kitsune!

Don't miss the over-the-top hilarity and subtle romance of this second volume of *Love Hina, the Novel.*

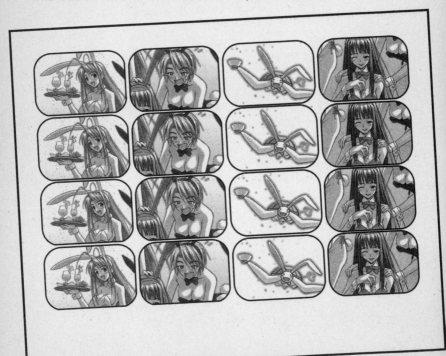

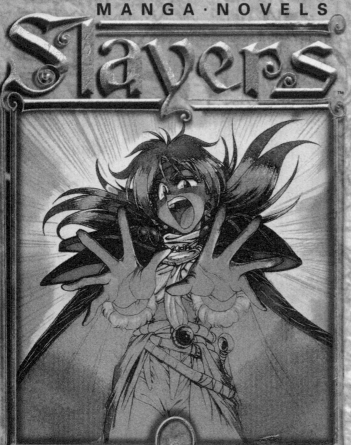

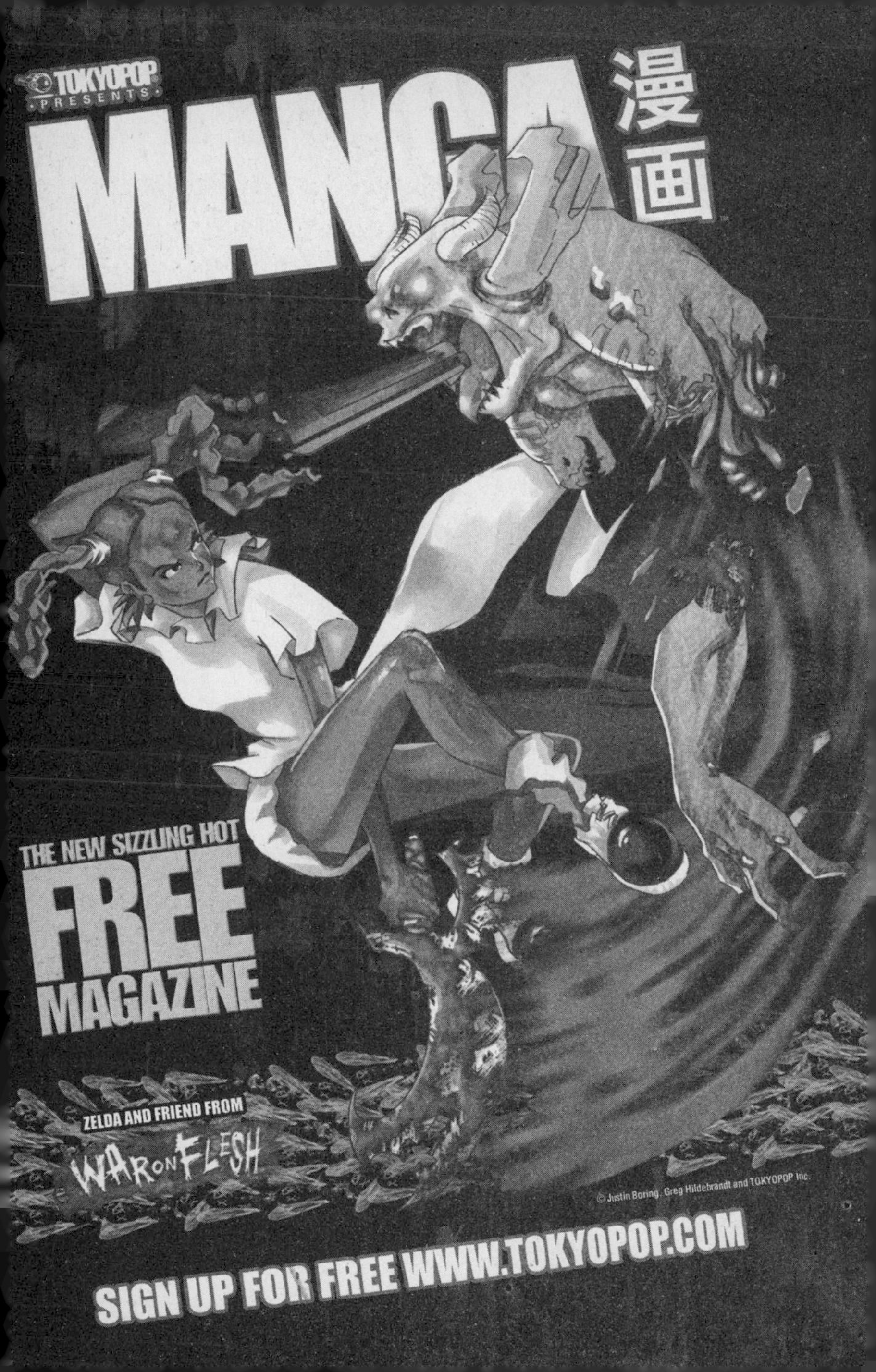
TOKYOPOP PRESENTS
MANGA 漫画
THE NEW SIZZLING HOT
FREE
MAGAZINE
ZELDA AND FRIEND FROM
WAR ON FLESH
© Justin Boring, Greg Hildebrandt and TOKYOPOP Inc.
SIGN UP FOR FREE WWW.TOKYOPOP.COM

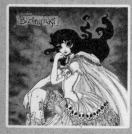
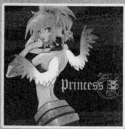

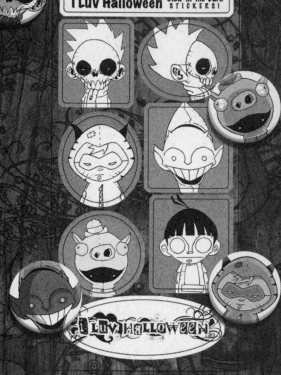

Music...mystery...and Murder!

RoadSong

Monty and Simon form the ultimate band on the run when they go on the lam to the seedy world of dive bars and broken-down dreams in the Midwest. There Monty and Simon must survive a walk on the wild side while trying to clear their names of a crime they did not commit! Will music save their mortal souls?

READ A CHAPTER OF THE MANGA ONLINE FOR FREE:

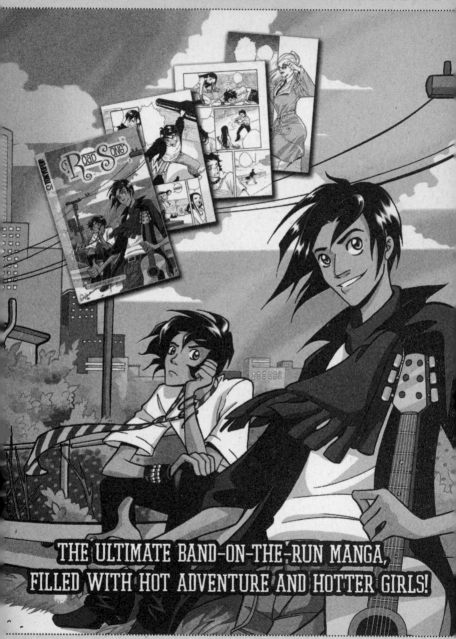

LIFE
BY KEIKO SUENOBU

Ordinary high school teenagers...
Except that they're not.

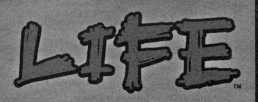

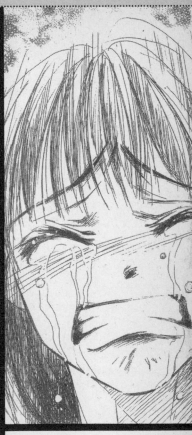

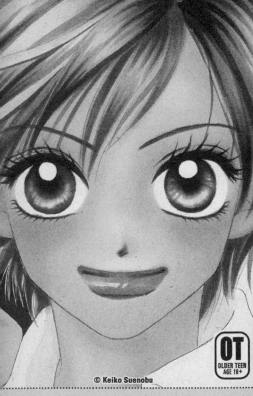

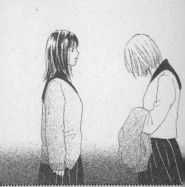

© Keiko Suenobu

READ THE ENTIRE FIRST CHAPTER ONLINE FOR FREE:

Ayumu struggles with her studies, and the all-important high school entrance exams are approaching. Fortunately, she has help from her best bud Shii-chan, who is at the top of the class. But when the test results come back, the friends are surprised: Ayumu surpasses Shii-chan's scores and gets into the school of her choice—without Shii-chan! Losing her friend is so painful for Ayumu that she starts cutting herself to ease her sorrow. Finally, Ayumu seeks comfort in a new friend, Manami. But will Manami prove to be the friend that Ayumu truly needs? Or will Ayumu continue down a dark path?

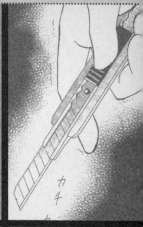

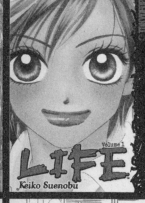

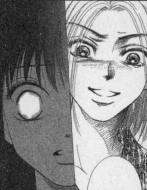

LIFE
Volume 1
Keiko Suenobu

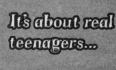

It's about real teenagers...

It's about real high school...

It's about real life.

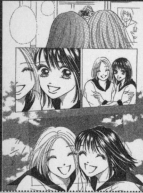

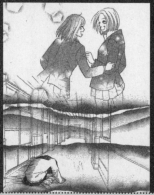

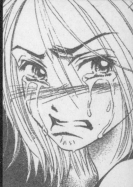

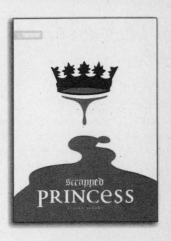
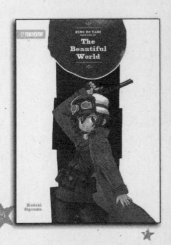

THIS FALL, TOKYOPOP CREATES A FRESH, NEW CHAPTER IN TEEN NOVELS...

For Adventurers...
Witches' Forest:
The Adventures of Duan Surk

By Mishio Fukazawa
Duan Surk is a 16-year-old Level 2 fighter who embarks on the quest of a lifetime—battling mythical creatures and outwitting evil sorceresses, all in an impossible rescue mission in the spooky Witches' Forest!

**BASED ON THE FAMOUS
FORTUNE QUEST WORLD**

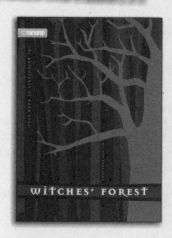

For Dreamers...
Magic Moon

By Wolfgang and Heike Hohlbein
Kim enters the enigmatic realm of Magic Moon, where he battles unthinkable monsters and fantastical creatures—in order to unravel the secret that keeps his sister locked in a coma.

**THE WORLDWIDE BESTSELLING FANTASY
THRILLOGY ARRIVES IN THE U.S.!**

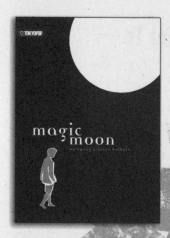

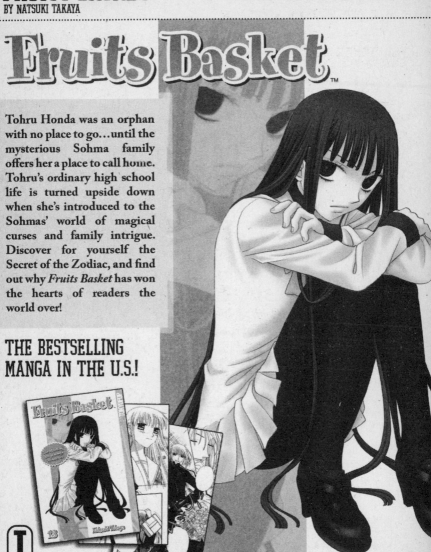

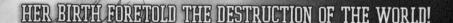